The Blood Cells
and Hematopoietic Tissues

The Blood Cells and Hematopoietic Tissues

Second Edition

Leon Weiss

Grace Lansing Lambert Professor of Cell Biology
Department of Animal Biology, University of Pennsylvania

Elsevier
New York • Amsterdam • Oxford

Text has been taken in total from *Histology: Cell and Tissue Biology*, fifth edition.
Leon Weiss, editor. New York: Elsevier Science Publishing Co., Inc., 1983.

Cover illustration is Figure 12-5.

Published by:

Elsevier Science Publishing Co., Inc.
52 Vanderbilt Avenue, New York, New York 10017

Sole distributors outside the United States and Canada:

Elsevier Science Publishers B.V.
P.O. Box 211, 1000 AE Amsterdam, The Netherlands

Library of Congress Cataloging in Publication Data

Weiss, Leon.
    The blood cells and hematopoietic tissues.

    Text consists of 7 chapters by Leon Weiss and taken from: Histology: cell and
    tissue biology/edited by Leon Weiss. 5th ed. c1983.

    Includes bibliographies and index.
    1. Hematopoietic system. 2. Blood cells. I. Histology. 5th ed. II. Title.
    [DNLM: 1. Blood cells—Cytology. 2. Blood cells—Physiology. 3. Hematopoietic
    system—Anatomy and histology. WH 100 W429b]
QM178.W45   1984   611'.0185   84-1621
ISBN 0-444-00926-4

Manufactured in the United States of America

Contents

Foreword

The textbook *Histology: Cell and Tissue Biology*, fifth edition, is a collaborative effort of thirty-three scientists to present to the student of medicine a comprehensive but manageable account of the structure and function of the tissues of the body. Because some readers will find certain chapters or groups of chapters useful but may not require the whole text, we are providing a number of monographs drawn from *Histology: Cell and Tissue Biology* and dealing with selected areas.

This book, THE BLOOD CELLS AND HEMATOPOIETIC TISSUES, consists of seven chapters on the blood and blood forming tissues written by Leon Weiss, the editor of *Histology*, fifth edition.

In order to expedite publication and to keep the monograph price as low as possible, all chapters have been reproduced exactly from the original negatives so that the original text —including references to other chapters—and the original pagination are retained. A new index has been added.

Preface

This book, consisting of chapters taken from the comprehensive textbook *Histology: Cell and Tissue Biology*, fifth edition, attempts to present an up-to-date account of the structure and function of the blood and major hematopoietic tissues. It depends heavily upon the morphologic techniques of light and electron microscopy, autoradiography, cytochemistry, and tissue culture as well as upon biochemical, physiological, and molecular biological methods as appropriate.

The functions of the hematopoietic system depend upon the cooperative actions of several cell types. Erythropoiesis involves macrophages, adventitial and endothelial cells of the venous vasculature, stem cells, and erythroblasts. Antibody production depends upon B cells, T cells, macrophages, and antigen-presenting cells. The development of blood cells, their migrations, and their sorting out in tissues depends upon interactions of stromal cells and blood cells. In these chapters I demonstrate that the structure of the hematopoietic system is the morphological expression of these cellular interactions and that without knowledge of its structure the hematopoietic system cannot be understood.

The textbook *Histology: Cell and Tissue Biology* for which these chapters were written is used primarily in the basic sciences—in courses in microscopic anatomy and in cell and tissue biology. Yet so interdependent have the basic and clinical sciences become that I believe the material in these chapters will be useful to clinical scholars specializing in hematology, immunology, and infectious diseases. This monograph is offered in an attempt to reach these clinical audiences.

I should like to express my appreciation to the Public Health Services for its support of research that is the basis of this monograph.

Leon Weiss

The Cell

Leon Weiss

General Properties

The cell is the unit of living structure. The tissues that form the body consist entirely of cells and of extracellular material elaborated by cells. The cell, moreover, can carry out an independent existence whereas none of its constituents can do so. Indeed, an entire phylum, the Protozoa, is unicellular, and isolated metazoan cells may be maintained in tissue culture.

Most mammalian cells are microscopic, although in some instances they reach macroscopic visibility. The limits of cell size are exemplified by bacteria or bacteria-like organisms, which may be less than 1 μm in their largest dimension, and by avian egg cells, measured in centimeters (Table 1–1).

A cell is a complex, aqueous gel made of protein, carbohydrate, fat, nucleic acids, and inorganic material. Protein alone or in combination with fat, as lipoprotein, or with carbohydrate, as glycoprotein, mucoprotein, or proteoglycan, constitutes the substantive structural element both of the cell and of extracellular substances. Enzymes, large molecules that catalyze metabolic reactions, are proteins. Products and secretions of cells may be proteins. Carbohydrate is the major source of energy in mammalian cells. Among the principal carbohydrates are glucose, a monomeric utilizable form, and glycogen, a polymeric storage form. Carbohydrates built into complexes with protein may play a role in linking cells together, are major components of extracellular tissues, are significant structural elements within cells, and serve as distinctive receptors on the cell surface. Fat, too, may be a source of energy to the cell. Moreover, fatty acids, which constitute the principal storage form of fat, provide the cell with efficient depots of energy. Lipids have major structural properties. Phospholipids and sphingolipids are important in the structure of biological membranes, making them preferentially permeable to fats; they also control the orientation and mobility of proteins in the membranes.

Inorganic materials occur in cells in a variety

of combinations. They may be associated with enzymes and with other proteins or fats, or they may be free of organic chemicals. They influence the adhesiveness and other physical properties of cells and extracellular materials in many different ways. Thus calcium contributes to the rigidity of bone; to the adhesiveness of the constituents of the subcellular particles, the ribosomes; to the capacity of cells to aggregate; and to the capacity of muscle to relax.

One of the achievements of microscopic anatomy is the ability to induce selective chemical reactions that reveal the location of different chemical moieties in tissue prepared for examination under the microscope. Chapter 2 is devoted to histochemistry, the term given to this division of histology, and histochemical findings are presented throughout this book.

There are two major classes of cells: prokaryotes and eukaryotes. *Prokaryotes*, exemplified by bacteria, contain nucleoprotein that may be segregated in the protoplasm as a *nuclear body* or *nucleoid* but is not enveloped in membrane. In *eukaryotes*, represented by fungi and higher forms, a true membrane-bounded nucleus is present. In fact, the eukaryotic cell is distinguished by well-developed membrane systems that not only envelope the nucleus but compartmentalize many cellular functions such as protein and steroid synthesis (the membranes of endoplasmic reticulum), respiration (the membranes of mitochondria), and secretion (the membranes of the Golgi complex).

The nucleus is typically a prominent ovoid structure lying near the center of the cell (Figs. 1–1 and 1–2). In it are chromosomes that contain *deoxyribonucleic acid (DNA)*, which encodes the genetic information. With the microscope, DNA appears as densely stained particles termed, in aggregate, *chromatin*. A nucleus may contain one or more *nucleoli*, typically spherical structures representing specialized modifications of chromosomes. There are several forms of a second type of nucleic acid, *ribonucleic acid (RNA)*. RNAs read the genetic code built into DNA and then play the central role in synthesizing the proteins encoded in the DNA. RNAs, themselves encoded in the DNA, are generated in the nucleus and are distributed in both nucleus and cytoplasm. Their complex structures and functions are discussed below.

The nucleus is surrounded by cytoplasm, the realm of protoplasm that expresses most differentiated cellular functions. The cytoplasm contains many highly organized, distinctive organ-

TABLE 1–1 Equivalent measurements

10 angstroms (Å) =	1 millimicrometer (mμm)
	or 1 nanometer (nm)
10,000 angstroms =	1 micrometer (μm)
1,000 microns =	1 millimeter (mm)
10 millimeters =	1 centimeter (cm)
100 centimeters =	1 meter (m)

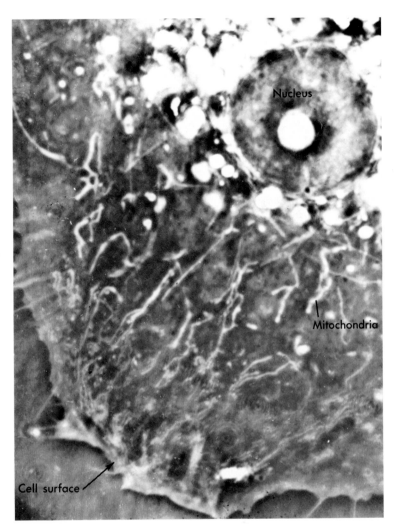

1-1 Hela cells, living in tissue culture; phase-contrast photomicrograph. Hela cells were derived by Dr. George Gey from a carcinoma of the uterine cervix explanted in tissue culture. They are maintained as a cell strain in tissue culture and used in a variety of experimental procedures. The cell border is ruffled and in places retracted, resulting in spinelike processes. The nucleus is spherical, surrounded by refractile clear bodies. Mitochondria are evident as irregular linear structures. × 1200. (From the work of Dr. G. Gey.)

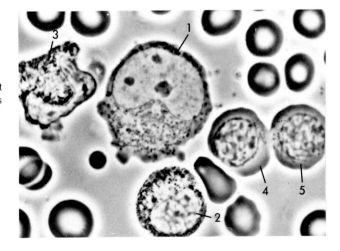

1-2 Human bone marrow cells, phase contrast microscopy. Developing white blood cells are present. They are myelocytes (1 and 2) and a metamyelocyte (3). Developing erythroblasts are also present (4 and 5) as are mature erythrocytes (unnumbered). See Chap. 12. × 1300. (From the work of G. A. Ackerman.)

4

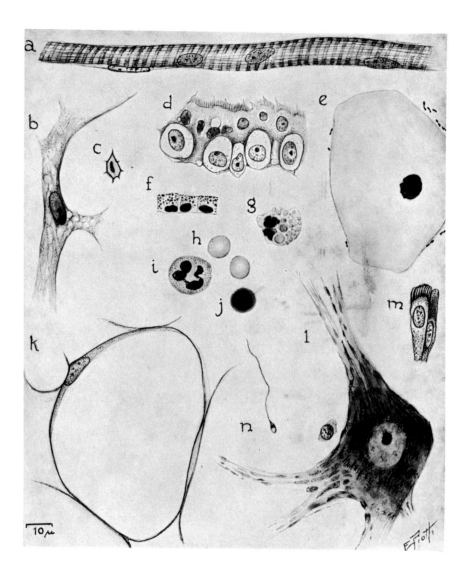

1–3 Variety of cells from the human body. **a,** portion of a striated muscle fiber. **b,** fibroblast from the umbilical cord. **c,** osteocyte within a bone lacuna. **d,** portion of the placental chorion, showing syncytial trophoblast and underlying cytotrophoblast cells. **e,** squamous epithelial cell and bacteria from a vaginal smear. **f,** three pigmented epithelial cells from the first layer of the retina. **g,** macrophage in bone marrow, which has ingested masses of blood pigments. **h,** two red blood cells. **i,** polymorphonuclear neutrophil; and **j,** small lymphocyte, all from a blood smear. **k,** fat cell from loose connective tissue. **l,** large motor neuron and adjacent small glial cell (process not revealed) from a hypoglossal nucleus in the medulla. **m,** adjacent ciliated and secretory epithelial cells from the oviduct. **n,** mature spermatozoon from semen. Cells a and d are multinucleate; g is binucleate; e has a pycnotic nucleus; c, f, j, and n have dense nuclei: the nucleus of l is extremely vesicular; i has a lobulated nucleus; the nuclei of a, g, and k are displaced by the cell contents. Some of the cells are rounded or polygonal, but a is extremely elongate, b and c have short processes, and the neuron in l has long processes (cut off here). The syncytium in d has a brush border; one cell in m has cilia; n has a flagellum. Cells a and l display cytoplasmic fibrils; f, pigment granules; g, phagocytized masses; l, specific granules; k, a space left by dissolved fat; j and the neuron in l, conspicuous amounts of cytoplasmic basophilia. [The diameter of the red blood cells (approximately 7.5 μm) provides a useful measure of the other cells.] All × 700. (Prepared by H. W. Deane and E. Piotti.)

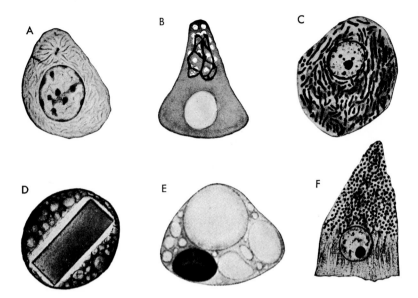

elles. These organelles include mitochondria, lysosomes, the Golgi apparatus, endoplasmic reticulum, centrioles, microtubules, microfilaments, ribosomes, secretory granules, and other structures that will be considered below. In addition, the cytoplasm contains such simple structures as glycosomes and lipid vacuoles. The cytoplasm is limited by a membrane called the *cell membrane*, *plasma membrane*, or *plasmalemma* (Figs. 1–2 to 1–5).

In metazoan or multicellular organisms, cells show marked specialization (Figs. 1–3 to 1–5). We speak of these cells as differentiated. In mammals cells vary in shape and size, exemplified by anucleate discoid pigmented blood cells 7 μm in diameter and branched nerve cells whose processes may reach a meter or more in length. Cell types may display pronounced internal variation. Striated muscle cells are packed with cross-banded filaments that slide on one another causing cellular contraction. Adipose cells are distended with fat, and secretory cells are filled with secretory granules. Osteoclasts may contain 25 or more nuclei, interstitial cells of the testis are packed with smooth endoplasmic reticulum, parietal cells of the stomach have rich infoldings of plasma membrane, renal tubular cells and brown fat contain extraordinarily large numbers of mitochondria, and immature erythrocytes are unusually rich in ribosomes. Keratinocytes in the skin may lose virtually all of their organelles and become scalelike structures packed with tough keratin filaments. So much has been

1–4 Various cytoplasmic organelles and cell inclusions. Because of their specific physical and chemical properties, these objects are not generally demonstrated by routine methods and are rarely revealed together. **A.** Cytocentrum in a cell of grasshopper testis, showing paired centrioles. **B.** Golgi material in a pancreatic cell of guinea pig, as demonstrated with osmic acid fixation. [Redrawn from Cowdry, E. V. (ed.) 1932. Special Cytology, 2d ed. New York: Paul B. Hoeber.] **C.** Mitochondria in a hepatocyte of a dog, stained with hematoxylin. (Weatherford.) **D.** Crystal within the nucleus of a hepatocyte of a dog. (Weatherford.) **E.** Spaces in a young fat cell left by dissolved fat. **F.** Secretory granules in a human pancreatic cell. Below and lateral to the nucleus lies ergastoplasm.

learned of the functions of the various cell constituents, in fact, that the function of a cell may be inferred from knowledge of its subcellular constituents. Indeed, such variations in cell structure and function constitute the backbone of this book.

The diversely differentiated cells that make up the complex metazoan body have clearly established a division of labor: the functions of the body are divided among them. Keratinocytes of the skin combine to form a tough protective barrier facing the outside environment. Erythrocytes of the blood, having developed chromoprotein pigment, carry the respiratory gases O_2 and CO_2. Muscle cells contract, nerve cells conduct, and bone cells provide a stable skeleton. The cells of the eye permit vision; those of the ear,

6

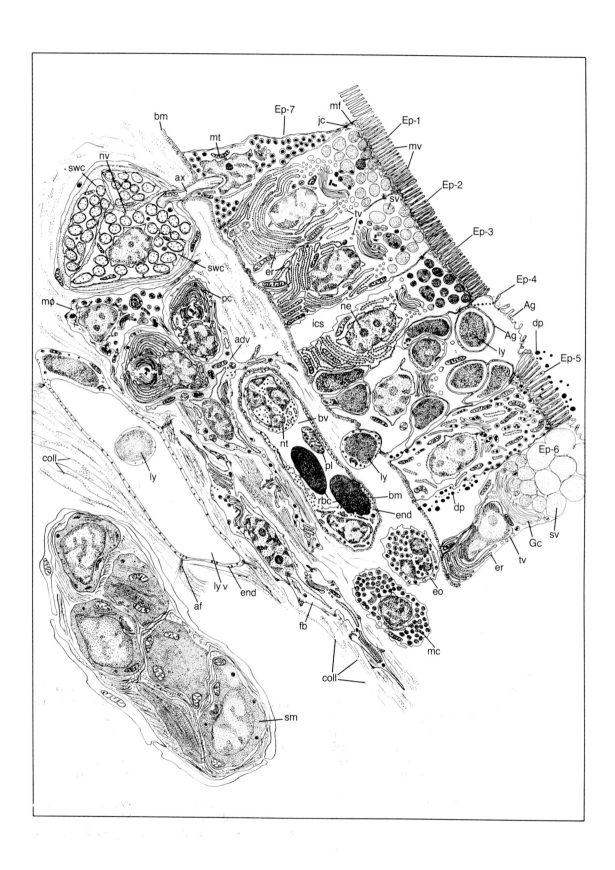

1–5 This drawing depicts a variety of cell types organized into an "imaginary" tissue that includes features of the gastrointestinal tract.

A major feature is the presence of epithelial cells lying side by side forming a surface that faces on a lumen. On their basal surface the epithelial cells rest upon a basement membrane **(bm)**. (Epithelium is discussed in Chap. 3.) These epithelial cells (Ep–1 to Ep–7) are bound together by junctional membranous complexes (Chap. 3) near their luminal or apical surface, while at their lateral surfaces below the junctional complexes **(jc)** the cells diverge somewhat, creating intercellular space **(ics)**. Epithelial cells Ep–1 to Ep–3 are secretory cells. They produce membrane-bounded secretory vesicles **(sv)** and release them at the luminal surface. These cells contain those cell organelles associated with secretion, viz: nucleoli **(ne)** euchromatin, endoplasmic reticulum **(er)**, transport vesicles **(tv)**, Golgi complex **(Gc)**, and condensing, storage, and secretory vesicles. See discussions of these organelles in this chapter and discussion of secretion in Chaps. 3, 20, and 21. The apical surface of each of these cells bear microvilli **(mv)**. Microfilaments **(mf)** form a terminal web beneath the microvilli and extend into them, conferring a contractile capacity upon them. Ep–5, also a secretory cell, produces mucous. Its secretory vesicles accumulate in the apical portion of the cell, but they are a good deal larger than those of Ep–1 to Ep–3 and they tend to coalesce. The Golgi complex is particularly well developed. Note that the outer nuclear membrane in the secretory cells is part of the endoplasmic reticulum and that the nuclear cisterna is dilated. The basal and lateral aspects of the cells may contain mitochondria **(m)**, which are often "pocketed" by infoldings of the basal and lateral plasma membrane. Ep–1 is an absorptive cell that takes up substances in the lumen, often modifying them, transports them across the cell, and releases them to the subjacent tissues where they may be metabolized or picked up by blood or lymphatic vessels and carried to metabolic centers such as the liver. Droplets **(dp)** at the luminal surface are taken through the microvillous border and enter the cell (endocytosis) in pinocytic vesicles (p. 52). These are conveyed to the lateral margin of the cell where they are released (exocytosis). They then travel extracellularly through the basement membrane to the subjacent connective tissue. Ep–4 is a highly specialized cell, the M cell, which is part of the immune system (Chap. 19). Lymphocytes **(ly)**, small immunologically competent cells that are responsible for such immunological processes as antibody formation, regularly enter and leave the M cell, lying in "pockets" of plasma membrane on its basal and lateral surfaces. The M cell takes up foreign material (antigen) from the lumen and conveys it, via pinocytotic vesicles, to the lymphocyte-containing pockets. M cells thereby present antigen to the lymphocytes initiating an immune response (Chap. 11). Ep–7 is a truncated epithelial cell resting upon the basement membrane but not reaching to the lumen. It contains granules that, on release, can influence the activity of nearby cells. A type of endocrine or paracrine cell, it may be part of the APUD system (see text). Note that it is penetrated by an axon **(ax)** that emerges from a small nerve **(nv)**. The nerve consists of a large cell, Schwann cell **(swc)**, whose cytoplasm carries many nerve fibers.

A stratum of connective tissue (Chap. 4) underlies the epithelium. It supports the epithelium and contains nerves, blood vessels **(bv)**, lymphatic vessels **(lyv)**, and free cells as macrophages **(mφ)**, plasma cells **(pc)**, fibroblasts **(fb)**, eosinophils **(eo)**, and mast cells **(mc)**. Connective tissue is characterized by abundant extracellular substance. This extracellular material often includes strong, supporting collagen fibers **(coll)**. The various cell types present in the connective tissues confer certain capacities on the tissue: plasma cells, antibody production; macrophages, phagocytosis; fibroblasts, collagen formation; eosinophils, phagocytosis, antiparasitic and antiinflammatory actions; mast cells, inflammation. Consult Chap. 4 (Connective Tissues) and Chap. 11 (Blood) for discussion. The blood vessel is a capillary whose wall is made of an endothelial cell **(end)** lying upon a basement membrane and an "outside" cell or adventitial cell **(adv)** (see Chap. 10). The capillary contains blood cells: a neutrophil **(nt)**, red cells **(rbc)**, and a platelet **(pl)**. The wall of the lymphatic capillary consists of endothelium alone **(end)**. The vessel contains a lymphocyte **(ly)** and its lumen is kept patent by the anchoring filaments **(af)** attached to the outside of the endothelium (Chap. 15).

Peripheral to the connective tissue layer is a fascicle of smooth muscle **(sm)**, which imparts contractile functions to the tissue.

hearing; those of kidney, excretion, and so on, as this book attempts to show. Implicit in such differentiation is the formation of tissues of diverse cells to effect these functions. Nerves conduct impulses, but they form a complex tissue. Included in this tissue are fibroblasts that produce collagen to support the nerve cells, glial cells to insulate them, endothelial cells to form blood vessels to carry blood to them, and other nerves to connect with them. Thus, specialized cells exist with other specialized cells forming specialized tissues that carry out specialized functions. The dominant or distinctive cells in such tissues are recognized as *parenchyma* (e.g., the nerve cells in nervous tissue) whereas the supporting cells can be designated as *stroma*. The *vasculature*, another essential "service" part of a tissue, may be included with the stroma.

It is further implicit in the existence of the diverse tissues working together to constitute a structurally and functionally coherent body that there are integrating systems. The classic integrating systems are the nervous system (Chap. 8) and the endocrine system (Chap. 21), which coordinate such complex events as reproduction, respiration, locomotion, etc. Histology is undergoing a revolution—no other term will do—because as additional actions of the classic systems are being newly discovered, hitherto unknown integrating systems are simultaneously being recognized. For example, a fair number of substances long known as regulators in other systems are now being uncovered as neural mediators as well. Prolactin, newly discovered as a central nervous system neurotransmitter has been known for years as a hormone produced in the pituitary gland and targeting the mammary glands where it induces the production and release of milk. There are, moreover, systems of *paracrine secretion* wherein peptides released by cells lying within a tissue govern the activity of other cells in that tissue. In contrast to the *endocrine system* in which hormones released from an endocrine organ typically travel some distance via the blood stream to reach a target organ, paracrine secretion is released and diffuses locally to affect local cells. Thus, paracrine cells in the epithelium of the gut release peptides that regulate motility, absorption, and secretion of nearby cells in the gut wall (Chap. 19). Some of these paracrine cells are fired by connecting nerves. A common characteristic of a subpopulation of such secretory cells in the gastrointestinal, respiratory, and several other systems is that they form their peptides or other low-molecular weight agents by taking up amine precursors and decarboxylating them. These types of cells have therefore been collectively termed the *APUD system* (*Amine Precursor Uptake and Decarboxylation*), further discussed in Chaps. 19 and 29. Still another network of cells with regulatory function is that of T lymphocytes, as discussed in Chaps. 11, 12, and 14. T lymphocytes have a controlling role over lymphocytes, macrophages, and related cells in inflammation and immune reactions. They may have a rather broad role in regulating cellular differentiation in other contexts.

Despite pronounced variations in cell structure, most cells do have much in common. Before exploring the general features of cells, we shall first consider some techniques widely used by morphologists.

Microscopy

In the most common types of microscopy of biological material, light or electrons are sent through a slice of tissue. The light or electrons are modified by the tissue as they pass through it. This modification contains information inherent in the specimen, and the function of the lens systems in any microscope is to amplify and convert that information to a form, an *image*, discernible by eye.

The human eye is sensitive to the contrast of light and dark and to differences in color. A light train may be represented as electromagnetic sine waves, color being a function of wavelength and intensity a function of amplitude. To render visible the disturbance in the light train induced by a biological preparation, the light must be modified in color or intensity. Some wave frequencies must be absorbed more than others so that the preparation will be seen to contain materials of different colors, or there must be a change in the amplitude of a wave so that the preparation will be seen to consist of dark and light parts. Thus, if the rim of a nucleus is darker than the surrounding structure, the nucleus is delineated and can be recognized (Figs. 1–3 and 1–4). If such structures as mitochondria or glycosomes can be distinctively colored, they can be recognized. Perhaps the primary role of the microscope is to permit the identification of different structures within tissues. Beyond such simple identification, however, there is considerable physical, chemical, and ultrastructural information inherent in tissues that can be revealed by specialized methods of microscopic analysis. These methods depend on various types of microscope, which we shall now consider.

Bright-field Microscopy

The bright-field microscope is a complex optical instrument consisting of three lens systems, a stage on which to place the preparation, and controls to permit focus.

The light is focused on the preparation by the condenser lens system. It passes through the specimen, where it is modified, and this modified beam enters the objective lens system. An image is formed in the focal plane of the objective. In that image lies whatever resolution the instrument is capable of providing. The bright-field microscope is theoretically capable of resolving points approximately 0.2 μm apart. The ocular or eyepiece then magnifies the image formed by the objective, presenting it to the eye as a visible magnified image.

The primary purpose in staining histological preparations is to induce differential absorption of light so that various structures may be seen in distinguishing colors. Staining has expanded from this elementary function until it has become possible to stain many chemical compounds selectively and specifically (Chap. 2).

Phase-contrast Microscopy

Although unstained tissue does not absorb light, it does affect light by retarding some wave trains more than others. Thus light may enter a specimen in phase, that is, with peaks and troughs of the component sine waves in register. However, the components of the specimen, having different optical densities, retard the sine waves differentially, putting them out of phase with one another. These phase differences are not perceivable by the eye. The function of the phase microscope is to convert phase differences into amplitude differences by matching the retarded waves with out-of-phase waves so as to cancel or diminish the amplitude of the retarded waves. The phase microscope thus permits one to observe considerable detail in unstained material and hence is suited to the study of living cells (Figs. 1–1 and 1–2).

Dark-field Microscopy

The dark-field microscope is also able to provide contrast in unstained material. Its effectiveness depends on excluding the central light train that comes into the objective from the condenser in the conventional bright-field microscope. Instead, the specimen is illuminated by light coming in from the side. Should there be objects of greater optical density than their surroundings in the field, such as bacteria moving in a fluid medium, they will deflect light into the microscopic objective and appear as light objects against a dark background. Little or no internal structure of the lighted particles is revealed. This technique has largely been superseded by phase-contrast microscopy.

Interference Microscopy

The interference microscope provides not only contrast in unstained preparations but additional information on the physical properties and the submicroscopic organization of tissue. Like the phase microscope, the interference microscope relies on phase differences induced in transmitted light by differences in optical densities in the parts of the biological preparation. However, the interference microscope is a quantitative instrument in which the light trains subject to phase retardation are compared with a reference beam. Because the optical density and phase retardation are in proportion to specimen mass, the mass of different components of the cell may be calculated.

Fluorescence Microscopy

The fluorescence microscope depends on exciting the emission of visible light in a specimen irradiated with ultraviolet light. Certain biological substances, such as vitamin A, are *autofluorescent*; that is, they can absorb light of one frequency and emit light of another. In practice, light within one frequency range, usually in the ultraviolet spectrum, is focused on the specimen, care being taken to protect the observer's eyes from this damaging radiation. This light is absorbed by certain structures in the specimen, which then emit light within the visible range, the wavelength of the emitted light depending on the chemical nature of the emitting substance. Although the autofluorescence of materials like

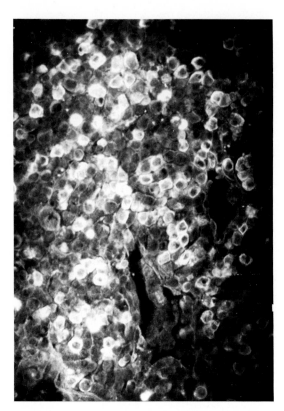

1–6 Fluorescence microscopy. A lymph node of a rabbit in the fourth day of a secondary antibody response to the antigen bovine serum albumin. The antibody, which has been tagged with a fluorescent tracer and is white in this photomicrograph, is present in the cytoplasm of plasma cells and lymphocytes. The nuclei are seldom stained and are present as negative (dark) images. See Chaps. 2 and 15. × 500. (From the work of A. H. Coons.)

vitamin A permits the use of this microscope with unstained material, the value of the technique is enormously enhanced by staining the tissue with fluorescent reagents (see Fig. 1–6 and Chaps. 2, 15, and 16).

Ultraviolet Microscopy

The ultraviolet microscope, like the fluorescence microscope, is built around the use of ultraviolet light instead of visible light. Its optical system is usually made of quartz, which efficiently transmits ultraviolet light. The image-bearing ultraviolet light coming from the ocular of the ultraviolet microscope is recorded on a photographic film, because ultraviolet light is both invisible and damaging to the eye. The value of the ultraviolet microscope lies in the fact that certain highly significant cellular structures, notably those containing nucleic acids, absorb ultraviolet light of specific wavelengths and can therefore be demonstrated. Because the wavelength of ultraviolet is shorter than that of visible light, this microscope offers somewhat higher resolution than the bright-field microscope.

Polarizing Microscopy

The polarizing microscope permits one to determine whether biological materials have different refractive indices along different optical axes. Such materials are *birefringent* or *anisotropic*. They are able to convert a beam of linear polarized light to elliptical polarized light, one axis of which can be transmitted by an analyzer and visualized. In the polarizing microscope, light is polarized below the stage of the microscope by a Nicol quartz prism or other suitable polarizer. The polarizer is made of material capable of transmitting only polarized light in one plane or axis. By rotating the analyzer, the polarization of the light transmitted by the specimen may be determined and any change from the character of polarization of the source detected. Substances incapable of affecting polarized light are termed *isotropic*. For biological material to change linear to elliptical polarized light, submicroscopic particles that are asymmetric must be present, and these particles must be oriented in an ordered nonrandom manner. Thus, the ability of biological material to change linear to elliptical polarized light indicates that its submicroscopic structure consists of oriented asymmetric molecules.

Filaments, fibers, and linear proteins are typically birefringent. Lipoprotein complexes, such as those composing membranes, may display complex polarizing properties. Typically, the orientation of the lipid molecules, and hence their rotation of polarized light, is at right angles to that of the protein component. Polarization optics have been fruitfully applied to the study of muscle, connective tissue fibers, cell membranes, and the achromatic mitotic apparatus (Fig. 1–7).

Transmission Electron Microscopy

The transmission electron microscope (TEM), in contrast to light microscopes, uses a beam of electrons in place of a beam of light. Additional

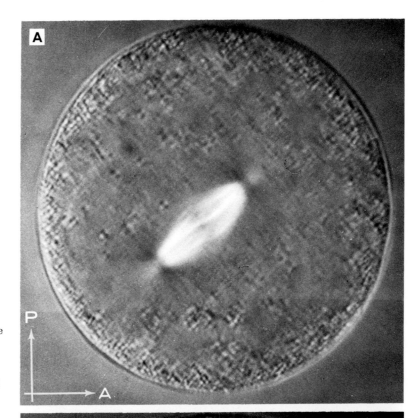

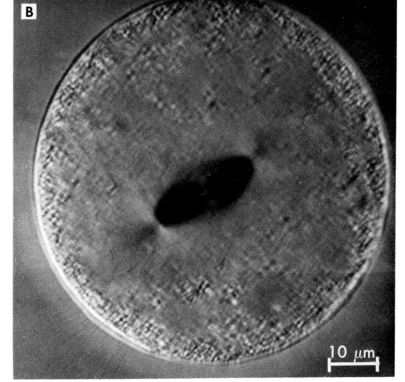

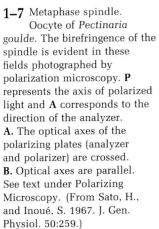

1–7 Metaphase spindle.
Oocyte of *Pectinaria goulde*. The birefringence of the spindle is evident in these fields photographed by polarization microscopy. **P** represents the axis of polarized light and **A** corresponds to the direction of the analyzer.
A. The optical axes of the polarizing plates (analyzer and polarizer) are crossed.
B. Optical axes are parallel. See text under Polarizing Microscopy. (From Sato, H., and Inoué, S. 1967. J. Gen. Physiol. 50:259.)

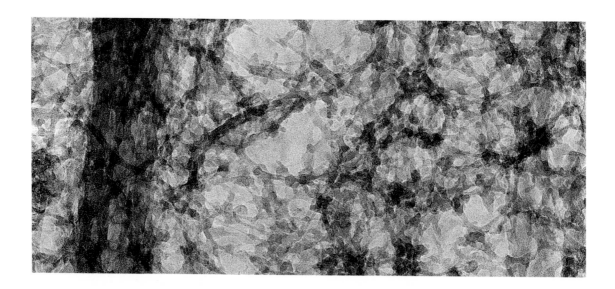

1–8 High-voltage electron micrograph. The electron beam, impelled at higher voltage, penetrates thicker sections and provides greater resolution than that in conventional transmission electron microscopes. This field includes the ground cytoplasm (hyaloplasm or cell sap). The ground substance of the cytoplasm contains a lattice of microtrabeculae. These form an irregular lattice which is continuous with the actin fibers (on the left) and support polysomes at their junction points. The microtrabeculae are about 30 to 50 Å in diameter and highly variable in length. The intertrabecular spaces provide for the rapid diffusion of water soluble metabolites. × 145,000. (Courtesy of John Wolosewick and Keith Porter.)

differences follow from the special properties of electrons. Electron beams are streams of negatively charged particles incapable of passing through glass. Hence, the lenses of an electron microscope are electromagnetic coils that surround the beam at different levels, somewhat like a set of collars. The strength of these electromagnetic lenses may be changed by varying the current passing through their coils. By varying the strength of the projector lens (the counterpart of the ocular of the light microscope), the magnification of the image formed by the objective lens is changed.

Electrons are charged particles, and because collision with charged molecules of air will absorb and deflect electrons and distort the beam, the optical system of an electron microscope must be evacuated of air. A vacuum of 10^{-4} mm Hg is commonly required. The electron stream is produced by heating a tungsten filament. The electrons are directed and impelled by moderately high voltage, usually ranging from 40,000 to 100,000 V. The higher voltages produce electron streams with shorter wavelengths, which are more penetrating and produce an image with less contrast but with higher resolution than lower voltages. Because electron beams are invisible to the eye, the images they form must be revealed by causing them to strike a fluorescent screen, and they are then recorded on a photographic plate.

Stability of the specimen is always a major consideration, and efforts must be made to protect the specimen against sublimation, distortion, and other damage by the electron beam or the vacuum. The specimen must be extremely thin for the electrons, so easily absorbed, to pass through it and create an image. Electron-microscopic sections are approximately 0.025 μm (250 Å) thick. Obtaining sections of tissues this thin has required the development of special slicing machines, *ultramicrotomes*, and a special technology of fixing and embedding tissues. Because thin sections have little intrinsic contrast, they must be stained with electron-absorbing heavy metals to provide the contrast necessary to reveal details of cell structure.

The value of the electron microscope lies in its great resolving power. Resolution of a microscope, measured as the distance between the closest two points it can distinguish as separate, depends on the wavelength of the radiation. An electron train has wave characteristics in addition to the characteristics of charge and mass. Its wavelength is small enough so that resolution of about 2 Å is possible and about 30 Å is routine. Consequently, a useful magnification of more than 500,000 is possible. The bright-field microscope, in contrast, has a resolution of approximately 0.2 μm and a useful magnification of 2,000. It has not yet proved practicable to examine living tissue by electron microscopy because of the vacuum and the damaging effects of electrons. Techniques that make it possible to obtain histochemical information at electron-microscopic resolutions have made electron microscopy increasingly productive. Moreover, quantitative analytic methods are available.

Variations on the TEM have been made. High-voltage electron microscopes capable of exceptionally high resolution exist. With accelerating voltages of a million electron-volts, they provide greater resolution and greater penetrating power of the electron beam and, therefore, the capacity to use thicker sections than is possible by conventional TEMs (Fig. 1–8).

Scanning Electron Microscopy

Scanning electron microscopy (SEM) provides a beautiful three-dimensional high-resolution image of cells and tissues (Figs. 1–9, 13–7, and 16–19). Moreover, cytochemical features can be localized on the image.

In SEM the surface of the tissue is studied. Whole mounts of tissue cultures or pieces of tissue are placed on the stage of the SEM. A slender electron beam or probe plays upon the surface, going back and forth in a regular way scanning the preparation. As the electron probe strikes the surface of the specimen, it generates several different kinds of signals. These signals include electrons (the so-called secondary electrons) and x rays. The secondary electrons may be focused on a cathode-ray tube or photographic film to form the three-dimensional image. X rays are generated when the electron probe strikes atoms having a mass greater than that of sodium. Each element is the source of x rays of distinctive wavelengths. The magnitude of the x rays generated is a function of the concentration of the element. Analysis of the x ray pattern of a tissue thus provides information on the concentration and distribution of elements.

Tissues prepared for SEM are fixed and dried. Drying at *critical point* has become the preferred method. The tissue is introduced into a suitable fluid and that fluid brought to its critical point, which is the combination of pressure and temperature at which the fluid and gaseous phases exist together without an interface or meniscus. Thus, there is no surface tension. The presence of surface tension during drying is disruptive to a tissue and causes visible distortions. After

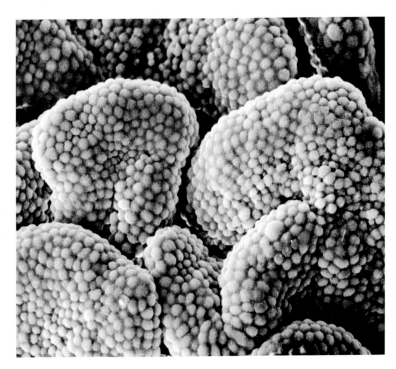

1–9 Scanning electron microscopy of the surface of the yolk sac. Note the three-dimensional character of the scanning electron micrograph. The surface is thrown up into folds, and each of the folds is beset with many cobblestonelike protuberances. The surface dips down around these protuberances. The appearance of this surface by light microscopy and transmission electron microscopy is presented in Chap. 27. (From King, B., Jr., and Enders, A. C. 1970. Am. J. Anat. 127:397.)

drying, the surface of the tissue is commonly coated in a vacuum with an electrically conductive coat of gold, gold–palladium, or carbon.

The SEM's resolution is inversely proportional to the diameter of the electron probe. Accordingly, SEMs possess very narrow, very coherent electron beams. Resolution of the SEM in the images generated by secondary electrons is 25 to 75 Å.

Biological Microscopic Preparations

Living Cells

Living cells may be maintained in tissue culture for long periods and examined by microscopy while undisturbed in culture. Tissue culture permits control of the environment and isolation of single cells or of *clones*, which are colonies derived from the proliferation of a single cell.

Maintaining cells in tissue culture requires considerable attention, involving nutritive media, control of atmospheric gases, and sterility. For short-term investigation, living cells such as leukocytes in a drop of blood may be placed on a clean slide, covered with a coverslip, sealed with petroleum jelly to prevent evaporation, placed on a warming stage, and studied under the microscope. This type of preparation is called *supravital* in distinction to more stable, longer-lasting preparations, such as whole animals or long-term tissue cultures, which are called *vital preparations*. Thus living cells may be observed with the conventional bright-field microscope or with the phase, interference, polarizing, or fluorescence microscopes. Living material may be studied unstained or it may be stained and remain alive, but such vital or supravital staining offers limited structural detail and damages the cells. Although it is valuable in special situations, as in the staining of the reticulocytes of the blood (Chap. 11), it is seldom used.

The nucleus, cytoplasm, mitochondria, Golgi apparatus, and centrioles may all be observed in the living state, as may such activities as motility of whole cells and the movement of structures within the cell.

The plasma membrane may be in active movement, associated with such processes as pinocytosis and phagocytosis (discussed under cytoplasmic vesicles, below). The study of living material offers certain satisfactions. Any scientific study induces artifacts, or departures from the natural state. A question that a scientist must always consider is whether or not the artifacts are consistent, repeatable, and significant—and therefore useful. Intuitively, one thinks that what is seen in the living cell is less apt to be an uncontrolled or misleading artifact and nearer to the typical, undisturbed life of the cell than what can be inferred from killed, sectioned, and stained tissue.

In order to obtain greater resolution and more chemical and other information about cells, it is necessary to kill them by fixation, section them into thin slices, and stain them. We shall now consider these procedures.

Fixation

Fixation is a procedure wherein a given cellular structure or activity is preserved or stabilized, often at the expense of other structures, for subsequent viewing with the microscope. Fixation is most commonly achieved by immersing the tissue in a solution of chemicals, but it may be accomplished by physical means, such as heat denaturation, freezing, or air drying. Although there are fixatives of general use, fixation may be quite selective. Thus, to study the structure of fat droplets, the tissues must be fixed in formaldehyde or other chemicals that stabilize the fat, and alcohol or other organic solvents that extract fats must be avoided. Fixatives that fix or coagulate protein are widely used because they preserve the general structure of nucleus and cytoplasm. Greater resolution and less distortion of cellular structures are obtained with a fixative that produces a fine coagulum than with one that produces a coarse one. Thus glutaraldehyde and osmium tetroxide, which cause a very fine precipitation of protein, permit high resolution without appreciable distortion of structure. They are the most widely used fixatives for electron microscopy. Phosphotungstic acid is a coarse protein precipitator that causes protoplasm to be thrown into heavy strands. For general work, therefore, it is used infrequently, but its drastic action may expose more reactive groups. More sulfhydryl groups are free to react after the coarse fixation with phosphotungstic acid than with fixatives that induce a finer coagulation of protein. For the special purpose of detecting sulfhydryl groups in tissue section, this otherwise unsatisfactory chemical may be the fixative of choice.

Fixation induces chemical change in tissue.

Thus fixatives containing heavy metals, such as Zenker's fluid, which contains mercuric chloride, may react with the carboxyl groups of tissue proteins and influence their subsequent staining. Aldehyde-containing fixatives, such as formaldehyde and gluteraldehyde, may react with amino groups in tissue and block them. Reagents such as bromine in the fixative may saturate double bonds and influence the stability and staining of lipids. Staining methods are available that detect enzyme activity. The fixative used for this purpose must be very gentle; most chemical fixatives tend to damage enzymes so much that they become inoperative and therefore undetectable.

Although fixation is commonly required in preparation for microscopic study, it must sometimes be avoided or its effects minimized because of unwanted chemical change. Some living tissues, such as a drop of blood or tissue cultures, lend themselves directly to microscopy and need not be fixed. The deleterious effects of fixation may be minimized by such maneuvers as freezing the tissue or using very dilute fixatives for very short times (see below and Chap. 2).

Embedding and Sectioning

After the tissue is fixed, it usually must be sectioned into sufficiently thin slices so that its details can be revealed by microscopy. Only in exceptional cases, as in spreading out a drop of blood on a slide, can the required thinness be obtained without slicing. The slices must be thin enough to transmit light (or electrons in electron microscopy). Moreover, since the depth of focus of microscopic objectives is shallow, clarity of detail is favored by thin sections. For light microscopy, section thickness varies from less than 1 μm to about 100 μm. Most preparations are about 5 μm thick. Slices this thin are made with an instrument known as a *microtome,* which consists of a chuck that holds the tissue, a knife, and an advance mechanism. However, tissue after fixation is often pulpy or brittle and impossible to cut into thin slices. It must be infiltrated with a stiff material that can be cut. Most of these infiltrating or embedding agents are fatty waxes, immiscible with the aqueous cytoplasm. Most fixing solutions, moreover, are aqueous. Therefore, to be embedded in the most commonly used embedding agents, which are paraffin or celloidin for light microscopy and the acrylic or epoxy resins for electron microscopy, the fixed tissues must be dehydrated. To this end the tissues are passed through a series of increasingly concentrated aqueous solutions of ethyl alcohol, acetone, or other dehydrating agents that are miscible with both water and fat. Thus the tissue may be passed through solutions of 50, 70, 80, and 95% ethanol, and then into absolute ethanol. Next, either directly or through an intermediate organic solvent like toluene, the tissue is placed in the embedding agent in a liquid phase. The embedding agent replaces the solvent and thoroughly infiltrates the tissue.

Paraffin is made fluid by temperatures above the melting point, usually about 60°C, and the dehydrated tissue is allowed to steep in molten paraffin. The preparation is then cooled. Having infiltrated the interstices of the tissue, the paraffin becomes solid, forming a block that can be cut.

In plastic embedding for electron or light microscopy, the plastic is introduced in the fluid monomeric state. With sufficient steeping, it infiltrates the tissue. Then, by means of heat or ultraviolet light, the plastic is polymerized and becomes, like paraffin, a solid in which the tissue lies thoroughly infiltrated and embedded.

However, a price must be paid to obtain such stable infiltrated blocks of tissue. The alcohols used to dehydrate tissues before infiltration extract fat, coagulate protein, and cause other chemical changes in a tissue. In order to infiltrate with paraffin, moreover, the tissue must be subjected to temperatures high enough to inactivate many enzymes. As plastic polymerizes, heat is given off and may damage the tissue. Paraffin and other embedding agents shrink and thereby distort the tissues. For these reasons, alternatives to these convenient types of embedding can be used. Water-soluble embedding agents are available that circumvent the need for dehydration so that fatty materials may be preserved.

Some enzymatic activities, however, are so fugitive that they do not withstand infiltration with an embedding agent. In such circumstances the tissue may be frozen, and the frozen block of tissue has the physical properties to permit sectioning. Freezing saves the time required for embedding. Tissues can be frozen and sections made, stained, and read in minutes, as is common practice in a surgical operating room.

Freeze-drying is a significant refinement over fixation by freezing or chemical means because it allows minimal distortion and displacement of tissues, minimal chemical extraction, and maximal preservation of enzyme activity for light microscopy. A small block of tissue is quick-frozen or quenched by immersion in isopentane in liquid nitrogen at a temperature of $-150°$ to $-160°C$. It is then placed in a vacuum and dried by sublimation of H_2O, thereby avoiding liquid H_2O, which causes displacement and extraction of cellular components. The dried tissue, while still in vacuo, may be infiltrated with molten paraffin.

In tissues that have been quenched, the sublimated water may be replaced by a chemical fixative in vapor form; this type of fixation is called *free substitution*. It offers the results of freeze-drying coupled with chemical fixation. An electron-microscopic technique, freeze-fracture-etch, has proved so valuable that it is described in detail below.

Mounting and Staining

After the tissue is sectioned for light microscopy, it is usually mounted on a glass slide and stained, although it is possible with phase-contrast or interference microscopy to study unstained tissue.

Freeze–Fracture–Etch

The technique of freeze-fracture-etch has become an invaluable method in cell biology for studying membranes (Figs. 1–10 to 1–14; Fig. 1–27). The technique avoids embedding and sectioning of tissue and may even avoid fixation. It demonstrates heterogeneity in biological membranes and illuminates the nature of cell junctions. Its applications have not been restricted to the study of membranes, however. Useful information has also been obtained on particles, filaments, ground substance within the cell, and extracellular substances. Freeze-fracture-etch depends on the rather simple fact that when a tissue is frozen and fractured, the fracture line tends to travel within membranes so as to separate them into inner and outer leaflets, thereby revealing structures previously hidden. This technique is carried out in steps (Table 1–2):

1. The tissue is removed from the body and fixed, although fixation may be eliminated.

2. After suitable rinses the tissue is transferred to glycerol. The glycerol infiltrates the tissue and protects against artifacts due to ice-crystal formation in the subsequent freezing.

3. The tissue is cut into small pieces and placed on metal (temperature conductive) discs.

4. The tissue is then plunged into a bath of isopentane, held in a temperature-conductive vessel partially immersed in liquid nitrogen. Temperature is low $(-160°C)$ so that the tissue is almost immediately quenched or frozen below the eutectic point of water. This is most important because it permits freezing without ice-crystal formation in glycerated tissue. As ice crystals form, they rotate and literally cut apart the tissue, causing visible artifacts.

5. The frozen tissue is quickly transferred to the chamber of a freeze–fracture–etch machine, where a number of operations can be carried out. The chamber can be cooled to a low temperature. It contains a razor on an adjustable swinging arm that can intersect the tissue. It can be pumped out to achieve high vacuum (approximately 10^{-8} mm of mercury). Moreover, it is equipped with platinum electrodes so that platinum can be evaporated to form a film over the specimen. Within the freeze–fracture–etch machine the tissue is maintained frozen and under vacuum through the production of a platinum replica (step 8).

6. The tissue, positioned on its disc, is now fractured by the razor blade on the swinging arm. The cutting edge of the blade strikes the tissue and starts a fracture rift. The free piece of tissue above the fracture flies off and is lost. The lower part of the tissue affixed to the disc now has an exposed fracture face. The face is relatively smooth, with glasslike frozen water surrounding the tissue and filling in the spaces between membranes, particles, and other cellular and extracellular structures.

7. The freshly fractured face of tissue is kept under vacuum for a short time, usually a matter of minutes. This represents the etching phase of the process, during which some of the frozen water at the fracture face sublimates into the vacuum. As a result, membranes, granules, and other cellular structures on the fractured surface now stand out in relief, the level of the frozen water table being below them.

8. Current is passed through the platinum electrodes and a layer of platinum is evaporated over the frozen-fracture-etched surface of the tissue. This platinum layer forms a tough membranous replica of the surface. The platinum is evaporated from a point source and reaches the tissue from a given direction. The platinum covers the tissue very much as snow falling from a certain direction covers a landscape. It piles up

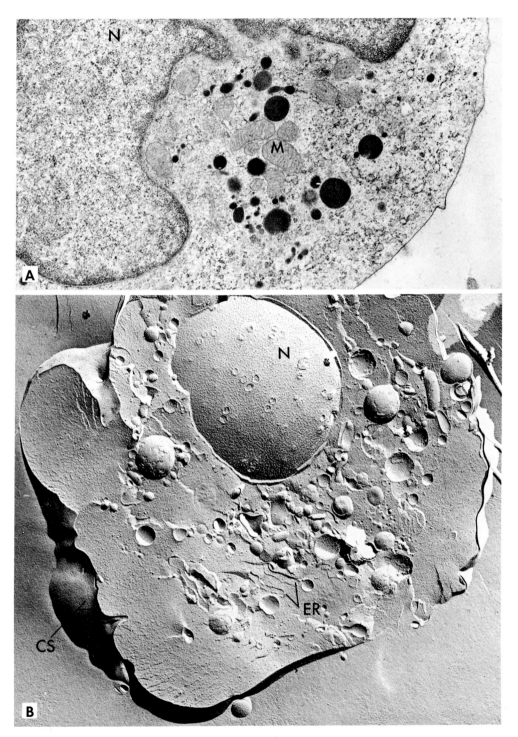

1-10 Guinea pig macrophage. **A,** A cell which has been fixed and sectioned and photographed in the electron microscope after staining with heavy metals. Nucleus **(N)**, mitochondria **(M)**, lysosomes **(L)**, and the plasma membrane are visible by this standard technique. × 13,500. **B,** A freeze-fractured-etched macrophage, showing the nucleus **(N)**, bearing nuclear pores, numerous globular profiles, two cisternae of the ER **(ER)**, and an invagination **(arrow)** at the cell surface **(CS)**, × 19,000. [From Daems, W. Th., and Brodero, R. *In* R. van Furth (ed.), Mononuclear Phagocytes. Philadelphia: F. A. Davis, p. 29.]

Table 1–2 Freeze–Fracture–Etch (Prepared by Dr. Maya Simionescu)

TISSUE FIXATION AND CRYOPROTECTION	FREEZING
1mm / 0.5 mm — 25% glycerol (diffuses into cells) / 4°C	tissue / forceps / carrier / freon -150°C / liquid N₂ (-190°C)
FRACTURING	ETCHING (optional)
knife / liquid N₂ / tissue / liquid N₂ -100°C / high vacuum	sublimation of ice / liquid N₂ -100°C / high vacuum
REPLICATION	CLEANING THE REPLICA
2 carbon backing / 1 platinum shadowing / liquid N₂ -100°C / high vacuum	strong bleach / replica to be examined by EM

on the near side of structures that rise from the surface and leaves a clear space or shadow on the far side. A carbon film is evaporated on the back of the platinum replica to strengthen it.

9. The vacuum is broken, the chamber is opened, and the disc bearing the tissue covered with a platinum replica is removed from the machine.

10. The replica is freed from the tissue by digesting the tissue away and is caught on a grid that fits into a TEM. Under the electron microscope, the grain of the platinum permits resolution to better than 30 Å.

Isolation of Whole Cells and Parts of Cells

Techniques are available for isolating cells from complex tissues and for disrupting cells to isolate their constituent parts.

A single cell type can be purified in a viable state from a complex tissue containing many cell types. For example, hepatocytes, the distinctive parenchymal cell type of liver, can be isolated from blood vessels, lymphatics, nerves, fibroblasts, macrophages, extracellular substances, and other cells and extracellular materials of the liver. The first step is to prepare a cell suspension of the tissue. In a few tissues, such as blood, this is not necessary, because the cells already are in suspension in the liquid plasma. In a solid tissue, however, such as the liver and kidney, the tissue is usually cut into pieces and subjected to enzyme digestion while it is shaken. *Trypsin*, a proteolytic enzyme produced by the pancreas, will digest virtually any protein substrate and is widely used in cell-separation procedures. With judicious application, extracellular substances will be destroyed or depolymerized and intercellular junctional complexes will be loosened without too much cell destruction. (A valuable related use of trypsin is for harvesting cells in tissue culture that are adherent to the flask walls. Brief treatment loosens the cells; overlong treatment digests and destroys them.) *Collagenase* is especially useful in freeing cells enmeshed in collagen. *Neuriminidase* can remove a sticky extrinsic carbohydrate, *sialic acid*, from the cell surface. (This example highlights a refined use of enzymes in cell biology in which certain receptors or other molecules can be specifically removed from the cell surface, such as *fucose* by *fucase*.)

After enzymatic treatment and mechanical agitation, a solid tissue is reduced to a suspension of diverse cell types and debris. A given cell type may be separated by one or more techniques. Cells will migrate differently in a countercurrent or in an electrophoretic system, and a given cell type may thereby be removed. In certain instances cells may be selectively eliminated, for example, by destroying erythrocytes with hypotonic solutions or destroying other cells with anticell antibodies. Cells may have different affinities for surfaces. If a suspension of macrophages and lymphocytes is poured through a column of glass wool, the macrophages will adhere to the glass fibers (from which they can later be removed) and the lymphocytes will go through. This technique may be refined by coating a surface with reactants that can hold certain cell types by interacting with specific cell surface receptors.

The major method for separating cells, however, is centrifugation, whereby the cells are subjected to pulls greater than gravity. (The number of gravities, or g, is a function of the speed of rotation and the distance from the center of rotation to the material in the centrifuge tube.) The rate at which a structure reaches the bottom of the centrifuge tube depends on its density and volume. Cells or other particles may thus be separated differentially by varying the time of centrifugation, with the denser and more voluminous structures coming down first. When centrifugation is complete, moreover, the larger denser structures are on the bottom of the tube and the smaller lighter ones lie on top of them. This is the technique of *differential centrifugation*. For example, the density of red cells is approximately 1.077 and that of white cells, 1.033. As a result, on differential centrifugation, the red cells and white cells are separated so that the red cells are below and the white cells above. (The sedimentation of red cell is enhanced by their tendency to aggregate into *rouleaux*, thereby increasing their effective unit volume.) However, separation may be cleaner by interposing a density barrier. That is, a suspension of blood cells may be layered carefully over a solution of bovine albumin or sucrose whose density is between that of red and white cells. The red cells go through the density barrier and the white cells do not, and hence a better separation is achieved. This is the principle of *density-gradient* separation. The technique may be refined by using a number of layers of varying density, or going gradually from low to high density without steps, resulting in continuous, or linear, density-gradient centrifugation. If the range of densities in such multiple or continuous density barriers encompasses the densities of the cells being centrifuged into them, the cells will come to rest in the layer whose density equals its own. This technique is *isopycnic centrifugation*.

In the separation and analysis of constituent parts of a cell, the main elements of the procedure are as follow. Fresh tissue is shred into small pieces or run through a grinder. Cells are then disrupted in a blender, or with a mortar and pestle, or ground by fine sand or in a mill by a closely fitting piston riding in a test tube. The tissue is thereby reduced to a pulpy heterogenous liquid containing disrupted cells and their constitutent parts, extracellular material, and debris. This homogenate is centrifuged and its different components are isolated. The nucleus is a relatively large, heavy structure and is concentrated in fields of low gravity. Mitochondria, ribosomes, lysosomes, and other cellular elements may also be separated differentially. An isolated component may be studied by electron microscopy to confirm its nature and to determine the damage done during its concentration and the cleanness of separation.

Microchemistry and Histochemistry

Microchemical methods developed as refinements of chemical methods. With them it has become possible to take a section of a tissue, study it with the microscope, and then take the section next to it and analyze it for inorganic salts, oxidative enzymes, or other components. It is possible, moreover, to dissect sections and carry out chemical analyses on small groups of similar cells or even on single cells.

Histochemistry, the visualization of chemical reactions in microscopic preparations, is so valuable that it is accorded a full chapter (Chap. 2).

The Structure of the Cell

Biological Membranes

Membranes are essential to cells. They are metabolically active sheets that enclose the cell as the plasma membrane. They also occur within the metazoan cell as nuclear membranes, endoplasmic reticulum, Golgi membranes, and as the membranes enclosing lysosomes, pinocytotic and phagocytic vacuoles, and many other structures. Membranes thus bound the cell and compartmentalize its elements. The organization and many of the functions of the cell, such as secretion of protein, synthesis of fat, detoxification of drugs, phagocytosis, respiration, and active transport depend on membranes.

The plasma membrane is the outer limit of the living cell and its face to the environment. It controls the ease with which substances enter the cell, providing it with selective permeability. The plasma membrane contains many and diverse molecules in its surface, which confer the capacity to interact with other cells and the extracellular environment. The fluidity of the membrane is determined by its ratio of cholesterol to phospholipid. Its permeability is also dependent on its lipid content. The membrane contains enzymatic pumps that control the levels of Na^+, K^+, Ca^{++}, and other ions both in the cell and its environment. It contains the enzyme adenosine triphosphatase (ATPase), which breaks down adenosine triphosphate (ATP) to the diphosphate (ADP), thereby providing energy for active transport (pumping), endocytosis, and other energy-costing membrane functions. (See discussion under Mitochondria.)

Some of the molecules that extend from the surface of the plasma membrane are *receptors* capable of selectively linking with substances outside the cell, including receptors on other cells. Many essential cell functions are receptor-mediated, such as conduction, phagocytosis, antibody production, antigen recognition, hormone-induced activities, and other cellular interactions in embryogenesis, cell homing, and cell sorting. Some receptors are shared by many cell types, such as insulin receptors needed in carbohydrate metabolism (Chap. 22). Other receptors are quite restricted to cell type, such as the *erythropoietin receptors* on erythroblasts, needed to capture the hormone *erythropoietin*, which drives the proliferation and differentiation of red cell precursors (Chap. 12). A cell type may show a succession of receptors as it differentiates, each stage of differentiation characterized by a distinctive set of cell surface receptors or markers, well exemplified by lymphocytes (Chaps. 11 and 14).

The phenomenon of *contact inhibition* is related to properties of the cell surface. Normal cells, as can be shown in tissue culture, cease to grow or move away when they establish contact with other cells; they show contact inhibition. Malignant cells, on the other hand, are not inhibited but move over other cells.

Most cells of the body contain an array of molecules on their surfaces, distinctive to cell type, encoded by major histocompatibility complex (MHC), the "supergene" on chromosome 6 in human beings that governs many cellular interactions, including immune-related actions (Chap. 12). Although not all of these MHC-determined molecules have been characterized or their formation determined, many of them seem to possess receptor functions. Cells, particularly those that are metabolically active, must literally bristle with surface molecules, an expression of the extraordinary importance of these molecules in regulating cell function. This discussion will be carried further after the chemistry and modeling of the plasma membrane are considered.

Plasma membranes, like other membranes, are complex and diverse. Their composition and functions have been studied by a number of techniques. They can be isolated by cell disruption followed by differential centrifugation and studied by x-ray diffraction, freeze-fracture-etch, and microchemistry. The erythrocyte plasma membrane has been extensively studied because large amounts can be easily prepared. As is the case with most membranes, it is preponderantly protein (50–60% of dry weight). This composition reflects high metabolic activity and structural stability. A notable exception is the lipid-

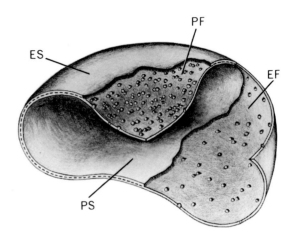

1–11 Diagrammatic representation of the four membrane "faces" that can be studied with the freeze-fracture-etch technique as shown on an erythrocyte. Note the terms used to designate the four surfaces: **ES**, the true outside surface of the plasma membrane; **PS**, the true inside surface of the plasma membrane; **PF**, the split surface of the plasma membrane which faces away from the cytoplasm; **EF**, the split surface of the plasma membrane which faces toward the cytoplasm. Particles, representing protein molecules, are shown only on faces PF and EF. (From Weinstein, R. S. 1974. The Red Blood Cell. New York: Academic Press, Inc., p. 247.)

rich membrane of myelinated nerves, whose high concentration of myelin appears to serve as an insulator. Most proteins associated with cell membranes are regarded as intrinsic to the membrane because they can be removed only by drastic procedures of extraction, digestion, or denaturation. The rest of the proteins are easily removed and thus considered extrinsic. Intrinsic or extrinsic proteins include structural proteins, enzymes, and receptor substances. Many of these proteins, notably the intrinsic ones, appear to be amphipathic, that is, asymmetric or polarized with hydrophilic groups at one pole and hydrophobic groups at the other. The implications of amphipathety are discussed below.

Lipids constitute 20 to 30% of the dry weight of erythrocyte membranes. Because lipid determines the permeability of plasma membrane, fat-soluble compounds readily enter cells, dissolving in the membrane, whereas fat-insoluble compounds enter by more complex mechanisms. The dominant lipid in the cell membrane is phospholipid, which is amphipathetic: the glycerol end is water-soluble, carrying phosphate and other ionized groups, whereas the fatty acid end is not, being lipid-soluble and hydrophobic. Other lipids include cholesterol and a minor component linked to protein or carbohydrate as lipoprotein or liposaccharide. Carbohydrate accounts for less then 10% of the weight of plasma membranes in most cells studied. It may be free as oligosaccharide or linked to protein or fat.

By TEM of sectioned tissue, the plasma membrane is approximately 75 Å in thickness with a range of about 60 to 90 Å. As with most intracellular membranes, it is seen as a trilaminar structure, termed the *unit membrane*, with outer darker lines approximately 20 Å wide and an inner lighter line, approximately 35 Å wide (Fig. 1–12). With high resolution, suggestions of bridges across the lucent central zone or of granular structures within the membrane may be present, but usually little or no specialization is evident. By negative staining some membranes, such as mitochondrial membranes, display distinctive structures (see below); but plasma membranes do not. A valuable technique in revealing structural heterogeneity in membranes is *freeze-fracture-etch* described above. By this method membranes are typically split into outer and inner leaflets, the split tending to occur in the central lucent zone (Figs. 1–11 and 1–14). As a result of this split there are four surfaces. The original surface facing to the exterior is the E *face* and the original surface facing to the interior, or protoplasm, of the cell is the P *face*. The fracture face on the exterior leaflet is the *EF* (Exterior Fracture) *face* while the fracture face on the interior leaflet is the *PF* (Protoplasmic Fracture) *face*. Particles may be seen on the split surfaces (Fig. 1–13). The number, size, and pattern of these particles differ from place to place in a given membrane and from membrane to membrane. By the use of labeled antibodies or other cytochemical procedures, it is evident that at least some of these particles are enzymes such as ATPase and adenylate cyclase.

A number of models for the organization of the plasma membrane have been put forth. That of Singer and Nicholson has received wide support (Fig. 1–14). Like other models, it postulates a lipid bilayer consisting primarily of phospholipid molecules oriented with their hydrophilic ends directed both to the outside and to the in-

1–12 Erythrocyte, peripheral cytoplasm. Note the trilaminar character of the plasmalemma, there being two dark laminae separated by a light one. This membrane is a unit membrane. × 280,000. (From the work of J. D. Robertson.)

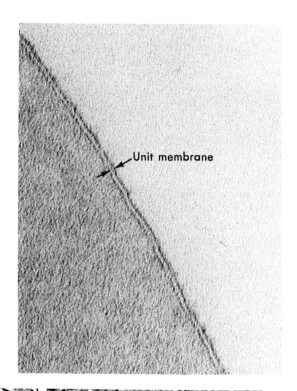

←Unit membrane

1–13 Replicas of freeze-fractured human red cell membranes. **A.** Freeze-fracture face PF originating from within the interior of the membrane shows more or less randomly distributed membrane-associated particles **(MAP)**, which may represent sites of integral membrane proteins. × 120,000. **B.** Face-EF has fewer MAP than face-PF. × 140,000. **C.** Freeze-etching has exposed the true exterior surface of the red cell membrane **(*)**, which appears barren and smooth. The fracture has entered the membrane **(arrows)** and exposed a PF-face for replication. × 100,000. **D.** Small fibrils **(arrows)** apparently extend from the cytoplasm of intact cells into the interior of the cell membrane. × 90,000. (From Weinstein, R. S. 1974. The Red Blood Cell. New York: Academic Press, Inc.) ▽

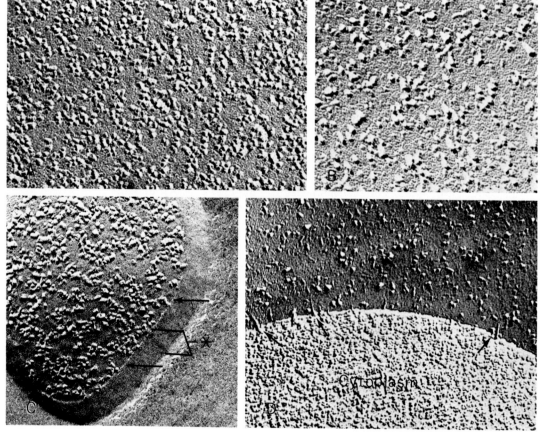

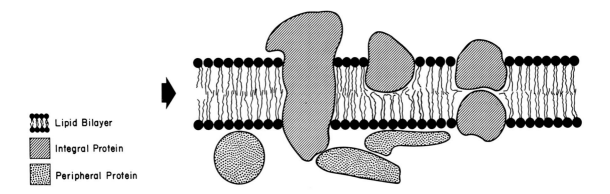

Lipid Bilayer

Integral Protein

Peripheral Protein

side surfaces. Being hydrophilic, the surfaces of the membrane interact with watery environments. Within the membrane, on the other hand, lie the long-chain nonpolar hydrocarbon portions of the fatty acid constituents of the phospholipid bilayer. The internum of the membrane is, therefore, fatty and hydrophobic. The phospholipid constituents of the outside and inside surfaces of the membrane, moreover, are somewhat different. Cholesterol molecules are dispersed throughout the membrane. Lying in the phospholipid bilayer like "icebergs in a lipid sea" are the proteins. They are most likely amphipathic with their hydrophobic ends lying within the membrane among the hydrophobic fatty acids and hydrophilic pole protruding from the outside or inside hydrophilic surface of the membrane. Certain intrinsic proteins are longer than the width of the membrane and therefore cross it, protruding from both inside and outside surfaces. These proteins are presumably hydrophilic at the ends and hydrophobic in the center. There are places in membranes, such as in the synaptosome of nerve and junctional complexes, unusually rich in proteins, which may be linked to one another. Proteins may be fixed in the membrane or may be rather loosely attached and move about in the plane of the membrane. Such movement can be demonstrated by an experiment in which certain receptors in the plasma membrane of mouse cells are stained with a fluorescent marker of one color and those of human cells stained with a fluorescent marker of another color. The plasma membranes, and thereby the cells, are then fused by the action of sendai virus. At first the labeled receptor substances remain apart, but within 40 min they appear completely intermixed. The mixing is temperature-dependent, occurring at physiological temperature but inhibited at 4°C. This temper-

1-14 Fluid mosaic model of cell membrane. The bulk of the phospholipids (**solid circles** represent polar head groups and **wavy lines** their fatty acid chains) are organized in a discontinuous lipid bilayer. Intrinsic or integral proteins are embedded in the bilayer but can protrude from the membrane. Extrinsic or peripheral proteins may bind to phospholipid polar head groups or to the membrane via protein-protein interactions. The **arrow** shows the position of the natural cleavage plane within the center of a lipid bilayer in freeze-fracture-etch techniques. (From Weinstein, R. S. 1974. The Red Blood Cell. New York: Academic Press, Inc., p. 239.)

ature-dependence suggests simple diffusion as the basis of mixing.

In addition to proteins intrinsic to the membrane, there are peripheral proteins, the extrinsic proteins, that are linked to the membrane. The contractile protein *actin* lies directly beneath the plasma membrane in microvilli and other places and appears linked to intrinsic proteins. As a result, the plasma membrane of the microvilli is moved when actin contracts. *Spectrin* is a linear structural protein that forms a bridgework beneath the plasma membrane of erythrocytes and inserts into the underside of the membrane. This membrane-associated protein both strengthens the plasma membrane, protecting it against the shearing forces of the circulation, and anchors many of those intrinsic membrane proteins that extend into the subjacent cytoplasm. Spectrin is in the class of structural filaments known as *intermediate filaments* (page 60). A further example of membrane-associated proteins are the *cytochromes*, which are rather loosely attached to the surface of the plasma membrane. Carbohydrates are often attached to the outside of the plasma membrane. Among them are sialic acid and other glyco- or mucoproteins. The carbohydrate-rich extrinsic coat may be so heavy as to be

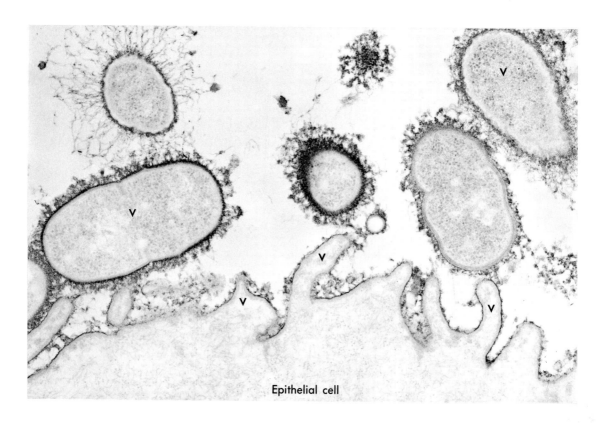

Epithelial cell

1–15 Cell surface, human buccal epithelium; electron micrograph. The free surface of an epithelial cell having large and small villi **(v)** is shown. A surface coat has been stained selectively with the dye ruthenium red. The coat, where it lies upon the plasmalemma, is relatively dense. On its free surface, on the other hand, the surface coat has a flocculent or filamentous character. × 40,000. (From Luft, John. 1971. Anat. Rec. 171:347.)

visible as a fuzzy layer called the *glycocalyx* and can be selectively stained by ruthenium red or lanthanum (Fig. 1–15). If sufficiently thick, it can be visible by light microscopy when stained by the periodic acid Schiff procedure. The sarcolemma of muscle and basal laminae in general may be regarded as sites of large-scale accumulation of proteoglycans extrinsic to the plasma membrane.

The Nucleus

The nucleus is the fundamental part of a cell that encodes the information from which the structure and function of the organism derive. The information is encoded in the genetic material DNA, complexed to simple basic proteins, histones, to form deoxyribonucleoprotein (DNP). With some exceptions, notably mitochondria, DNA lies exclusively in the nucleus. DNA is capable of replicating itself, thereby providing precise copies of the genetic code that are passed on to daughter cells by cellular division.

The nucleus also plays a central role in synthesizing proteins and polypeptides from the genetic information it carries. All the nucleated cells of the body contain the same genes, yet cells differ in their structure, function, and products. The nucleus differentially controls the use of this information from cell to cell by repressing or derepressing the action of various genes. The nucleus initiates the translation of its encoded information into the synthesis of proteins by mean of RNAs, a group of nucleic acids that differ from DNA primarily in base composition. Some RNAs are complexed to proteins to form ribonucleoprotein (RNP). The RNAs are produced in or under the control of the nucleus and are released to the cytoplasm where they engage in protein synthesis. The "machine" that assembles proteins from amino acids is a complex of RNAs and protein, the *ribosome*, whose constituents are produced in a nuclear component, the *nucleolus*. Other RNAs are *messenger RNA* (mRNA), which links ribosomes into working units called *polyribosomes*, and *transfer RNA* (tRNA), which carries amino acids to the polyribosomes to initiate protein synthesis.

A nucleus is present in virtually all differentiated metazoan cells, being absent only from mammalian erythrocytes and a few other end-stage cell types. Certain cell types have many nuclei or are polyploid (see below); the number of genes and other elements in the protein-synthesizing apparatus of a cell is thus multiplied and the cell is able to produce a greater volume of product. Hepatocytes, particularly with age, may develop two or more nuclei, and renal tubular cells may be binucleate. Osteoclasts or foreign-body giant cells may contain 25 or more nuclei. A mechanism for increasing nuclear function without increasing nuclear number is polyploidy, an increase in the number of chromosomal pairs within a single nucleus. Most somatic cells are diploid (2n), having one pair of each chromosome characterizing its species, but cells may develop two pairs (4n) or more. Hepatocytes tend to increase in ploidy with age; in old rats they are often 8n and 16n. Megakaryocytes, giant cells of the bone marrow containing a giant polymorphous nucleus may become 32n or 64n. A more restricted mechanism for increasing nuclear components is an increase in the number of nucleoli in certain oocytes, with a concomitant increase in production of ribosomal RNA.

The nucleus may occur in a dividing (mitotic or meiotic) state, during which it reproduces itself, or in a nondividing or interphase state. The interphase nucleus is most frequently encountered, because nuclear division takes approximately 1 h whereas, even in actively dividing cells, 6 h or more elapse between divisions. Many cells of the body seldom divide (e.g., hepatocytes) or never divide (e.g. nerve cells). (See section below on Life Cycle of Cells.)

In most cell types the interphase nucleus is an ovoid structure several micrometers in diameter (Figs. 1–10 and 1–16 to 1–18). In the leukocytes of blood and connective tissues, the nucleus is lobulated and hence termed polymorphous (see Chaps. 11 and 12). The nucleus is deformable and may therefore be pressed into a reniform or horseshoe shape. In contracted smooth muscle, it may be twisted like a corkscrew (Fig. 1–18).

The interphase nucleus is bounded by a nu-clear envelope and typically contains several distinctive structures. These structures include chromatin, nuclear sap or karyolymph, and one or more nucleoli. The protoplasm of the nucleus is termed *nucleoplasm* or *karyoplasm*.

Chromatin. Chromatin, by light microscopy, consists of irregular clumps or masses that, although not highly constant, tend to be characteristic in texture, quantity, and size for any given cell type. These clumps, sometimes called *karyosomes*, have an affinity for basic dye because chromatin contains DNA. DNA confers distinctive staining reactions on chromatin. Thus, chromatin is specifically stained in the Feulgen reaction. It selectively binds methyl green. In Romanovsky preparations, which are stained with methylene blue and azures, chromatin is stained violet (Chap. 11). These distinctive DNA staining reactions are abolished by pretreating the specimen with the enzyme *deoxyribonuclease*.

Chromatin is the embodiment in the interphase nucleus of the DNP of chromosomes. The chromosomes in the interphase nucleus are very slender, long, threadlike structures lying in a rather tangled mass. It is impossible to delineate individual chromosomes from this tangle. Indeed, it was at one time thought that this mass was a continuous single thread instead of individual interlaced chromosomes, and the name *spireme* was applied to it.

Chromosomes may be either coiled or uncoiled along their length. Whenever the tight coiling of the chromosome forms clumps greater than 0.2 μm in dimension, they are visible with the light microscope. Chromosomes in this form constitute the *heterochromatin*. The karyosomes are heterochromatin. In many cells, moreover, heterochromatin is also applied against the inner surface of the nuclear envelope, forming an outer rim of the nucleus interrupted only by nuclear pores (Figs. 1–10, and 1–17 to 1–19). There is also nuclear membrane–associated chromatin. Because the chromatin in uncoiled chromosomes, the *euchromatin*, is below the limit of resolution of the light microscope, euchromatin is "invisible" and cannot be differentiated from the nuclear sap. The proportions of euchromatin and heterochromatin and the distribution of heterochromatin can be quite characteristic for a given cell type. In fact, in the interphase nucleus, chromosomes may be tightly coiled in certain segments and uncoiled in other segments. Cells

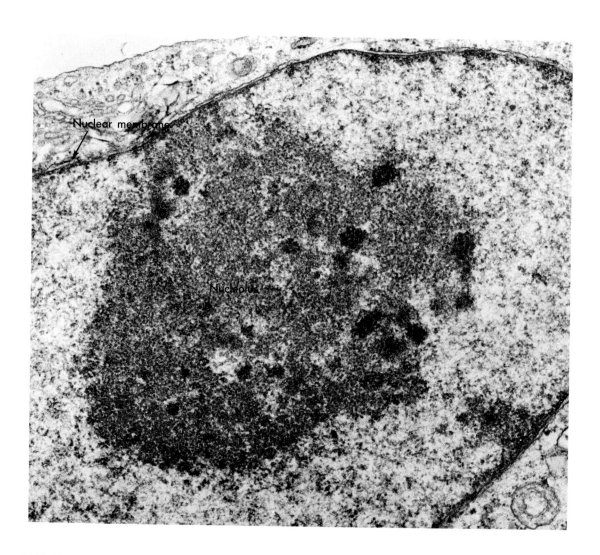

1–16 Rhesus kidney cell (strain MA 104) in culture.
The nucleolus, stained with uranyl acetate and lead, is well developed. It touches the inside surface of the nuclear membrane. Heterochromatin, densely stained, is present as a rim against the inside surface of the inner nuclear membrane. Most of the chromatin is dispersed and presents as euchromatin. The outer nuclear membrane (nuclear membrane) stands out clearly. It is part of the endoplasmic reticulum and, at places, bears ribosomes on its surface. See Fig. 1–25. × 40,000. (From the work of A. Monneran.)

with large blocks of heterochromatin tend to be relatively inactive in an early stage of protein synthesis, the production of mRNA. The uncoiled chromosomes are in the functional state that enables transcription of DNA through the formation of mRNA. The uncoiled chromosomes

serve as a *template* for transcription of information to mRNA. This messenger leaves the nucleus and enters the cytoplasm. There, in concert with tRNA and the ribosomal RNA (rRNA) of the ribosomes, it synthesizes proteins whose structure was encoded in the DNA. Thus cells whose nuclei are relatively rich in euchromatin tend to be quite active in the transcription phase of protein synthesis. In cells of females a characteristic mass of heterochromatin lying against the nuclear membrane represents one of the female sex chromosomes, an X chromosome, which remains tightly coiled through interphase. It is called *sex chromatin* or, after its discoverer, the *Barr body* (Fig. 1–20). It enables the genetic sex of an individual to be determined, a procedure of value in certain endocrinopathies or congenital disturbances in which the genetic sex may not be ap-

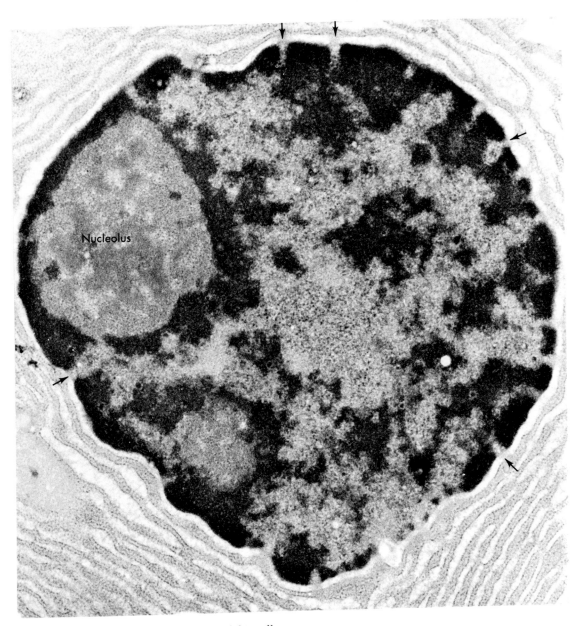

1–17 Pancreatic acinar cell. The nucleus of this cell, which secretes digestive enzymes, has been selectively treated to enhance the staining of DNA and to reduce the staining of the nucleoli and other RNA-containing structures. Chromatin is densely stained. Much of it is marginated on the inner surface of the nuclear membrane. Nuclear pores are prominent **(arrow)**, their location marked by the lightly stained aisles between heterochromatin masses. The section was treated with picric acid, uranyl acetate, and lead. × 30,000. (From the work of A. Monneron.)

1–18 Contracted muscle cell. The nucleus has been twisted into a corkscrew spiral. On relaxation, the nucleus will untwist and be cigar-shaped.

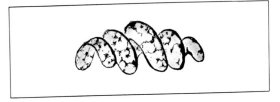

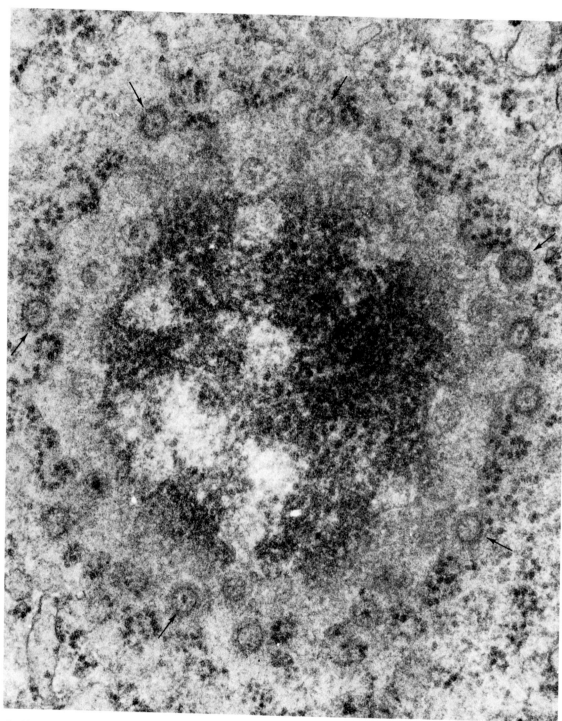

1–19 Rat hepatocyte. This is a tangential section of the nucleus, revealing nuclear pores all around **(arrow),** some with a dark central granule. Note that polyribosomes are in close association with the pores. This preparation is stained with uranyl acetate and lead. × 140,000. (From the work of A. Monneron.)

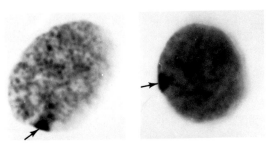

1-20 Sex chromatin of a human female. The chromatin lies against the nuclear membrane **(arrows).** This formation of sex chromatin appears to be due to the persistent coiling in interphase in one of the X chromosomes. Human buccal mucosa. × 4000. (From the work of B. R. Migeon.)

parent. The Y (male) chromosome may be demonstrated in interphase nuclei by a special fluorescence staining method.

The elements of the interphase nucleus—namely, chromatin, nucleoli (see below), karyolymph, and nuclear membranes—are readily identified by electron microscopy. However, the correlation of electron-microscopic observations of interphase nuclei with what is inferred of the structure of chromosomes and other nuclear components from genetic and other data remains rudimentary. It is known, for example, that an uncoiled chromosome may be of the order of 10,000 times the largest dimension of the nucleus. But it is difficult to gain any appreciation from sections of nuclei of the nature of the immense folding and coiling that the chromosomes must undergo. Such inferences as electron microscopy affords come from preparations in which chromosomes are floated out of disrupted nuclei, dried down on supporting membranes, and examined whole. In these preparations high degrees of coiling and folding are evident. Pure DNA may be prepared and examined as whole, unsectioned filaments by electron microscopy. These filaments are approximately 20 Å in diameter. DNA can be identified in sectioned interphase nuclei on the basis of selective staining. It is present in filaments of varying diameter, that of the slimmest being about 100 Å. The greater thickness of DNA in sections may be due to such factors as coiling, folding, or intertwining of DNA filaments or complexing of DNA with histones or other substances.

Nucleolus. A nucleolus is a discrete intranuclear structure consisting largely of protein and RNA, which synthesizes the major components of ribosomes. The nucleolus is well developed in cells active in protein synthesis. Such cells may contain several nucleoli. In cells synthesizing little protein, such as spermatocytes, neutrophils, and muscle cells, a nucleolus may not be evident. Nucleoli appear at certain specific sites, the *nucleolar organizing sites* in certain chromosomes (Fig. 1-21). These sites represent secondary constrictions in the chromosomes. At these sites on the chromosomes, the gene sequences *(cistrons)* are located that encode the genetic information for the synthesis of rRNA. Nucleoli remain attached to the chromosomes at nucleolar organizing sites.

Nucleoli by light microscopy are usually spherical, up to 1 μm in diameter, but may be oval or even bow-tie shaped. They are usually compact and sharply outlined, but they may be porous with fuzzy borders. Nucleoli may lie at random or against the inside of the nuclear membrane, an efficient location for discharging substances into the cytoplasm (Figs. 1-3 and 1-4).

Nucleoli are rich in RNA. Thus they absorb ultraviolet light at a wavelength of 2,600 Å, and can thereby be identified by ultraviolet microscopy. Nucleoli may be stained with pyronin in the methyl green-pyronin mixture and blue in Romanovsky blood stains. Staining of nucleoli is abolished by treating the section with *ribonu-*

1-21 Chromosomes containing nucleolar organizing sites from the clawed toad *Xenopus laevis.* They are taken from the metaphase karyotype (see text). Each of the chromosomes in the wild type contains very slender zones, the nucleolar organizing sites. In the heterozygote, on the other hand, only one pair of chromosomes contains this site. The resultant heterozygote, as discussed in the text, is nucleolar-deficient mutants. (From the work of D. D. Brown.)

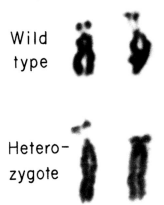

Wild type

Hetero- zygote

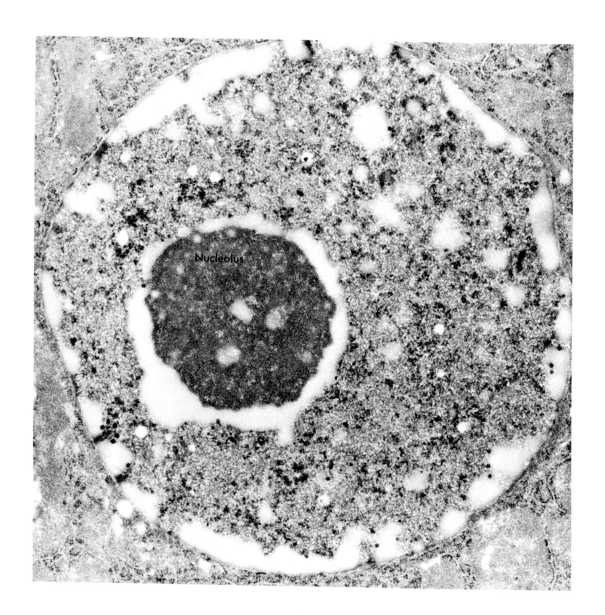

1–22 Hepatocyte. In this preparation RNP is preferentially stained and chromatin is bleached. The nucleolus stands out sharply. Stained granules, presumably containing RNA, lie outside the nucleolus in association with the chromatin. There are large (400 to 500 Å) perichromatin granules and small (200 Å) interchromatin granules. × 27,000. (From the work of A. Monneron; see also Bernhard, W. 1969. J. Ultrastruct. Res. 27:250.)

clease. RNA contains the nucleotide base *uridine.* (*Thymidine* is the DNA base counterpart to uridine.) Therefore, if radioactive uridine is given to an animal, autoradiography of its cells shows positive nucleoli (Fig. 1–23).

By electron microscopy, nucleoli contain two forms of RNA (Figs. 1–16, 1–17, 1–22, and 1–23). One is granular, approximately 150 Å in diameter, and represents maturing forms of RNP particles. This is typically the dominant nucleolar structure. The second form of RNA is fibrillar, 50 to 80 Å in thickness, and is probably a precursor to the granules.

Nucleoli are not the only sites of RNP in the nucleus. Particles of different sizes and filaments of RNP lie against and between chromatin. It is likely that some of this widely dispersed nuclear RNA is mRNA (see below) produced on extended segments of DNA (euchromatin).

DNA is a component of the nucleolus, desig-

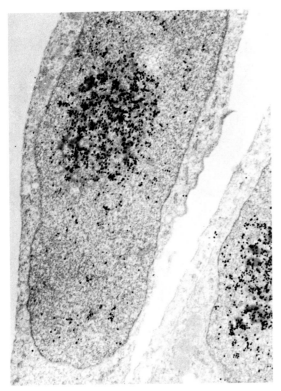

1–23 Monkey kidney cells (strain BSC). These cells,
in tissue culture, were exposed to [³H] uridine
(a precursor of RNA) for 30 min and then fixed and
processed for EM autoradiography. The distribution of
silver grains is only over the nucleus and mainly over
the nucleolus. ×25,000. (From A. Monneron, J.
Burglen, and W. Bernhard. 1970. J. Ultrastruct. Res.
32:370.)

nated *nucleolar chromatin* of the nucleolar organizing site of the chromosome. It occurs in
twisted or single filaments 200 to 300 Å in diameter.

Poorly defined granular material, probably
protein, occurs throughout nucleoli. Rarefied
vacuolar zones, not membrane-bounded, may be
present.

The nucleolus is a center for the synthesis of
ribosomes. The size and number of nucleoli depend on the level of rRNA synthesis. In actively
secretory cells (pancreatic acinar cells) nucleoli
are large and multiple, whereas in cells showing
a low level of protein synthesis (muscle cells,
certain small lymphocytes) nucleoli may be
small or absent.

Ribosomes have several subunits (see section
on Ribosomes). On the basis of isolation and
sedimentation analysis it appears that nucleoli

produce the subunits of ribosomes and release
them to the cytoplasm. The release to the cytoplasm may be facilitated by the nucleolus moving against the nuclear membrane and discharging through nuclear pores. In the cytoplasm, the
nucleolar-produced ribosomal components may
mature further, perhaps by adding protein, and
combine to form ribosomes.

Support for the role of nucleoli in ribosomal
synthesis comes from the work of Brown and his
associates on amphibian mutants lacking nucleoli. The embryo of the clawed toad *Xenopus
laevis* synthesizes few ribosomes before the tail
bud stage, the ribosomes from the oocyte serving
until that time. A lethal anucleolate mutant of
Xenopus may be bred from a spontaneously occurring heterozygote mutant with but one nucleolus per cell, instead of the normal two. Development of the anucleolate embryos is retarded
after hatching. The embryos are microcephalic
and edematous and die before feeding. The mutation that prevents the formation of a normal
nucleolus also prevents synthesis of 28S and 18S
rRNA, as well as high molecular-weight precursor molecules of ribosomes.

The correlation between ribosome production
and nucleoli is evident in multinucleolate
amphibian oocytes where the DNA specify-
ing the sequences for 28S and 18S rRNAs is selectively replicated. As many as 1,000 auton-
omously functional nucleoli may occur per
oocyte (Fig. 1–24).

1–24 Nucleus isolated from an oocyte of *Xenopus
laevis*. The nucleus was dissected from the
oocyte, flooded with cresyl violet stain, and
photographed. The deeply stained spots are those of
the hundreds of nucleoli which are in the plane of
focus. (From Brown, D. D., and Dawid, I. B. 1968.
Science 160:272.)

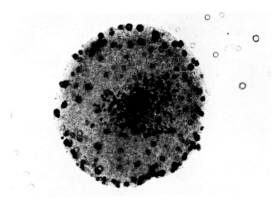

Nuclear Envelope. The nuclear envelope consists of two concentric unit membranes (Fig. 1–5). Each is approximately 70 Å in thickness, the inner one somewhat thinner. The space of the cisterna between inner and outer nuclear membranes varies in size and content. It is commonly about 150 Å wide and lucent. The outer nuclear membrane is continuous with the endoplasmic reticulum (ER), both rough and smooth. The cytoplasmic character of nuclear membrane is underscored in reformation in the telophase. The nuclear membranes are clearly formed by segments of ER, which line up around the reconstituted nuclear mass. In cells synthesizing protein, the nuclear envelope may, like the rough ER, contain the protein product. Thus, in antibody-producing cells the nuclear envelope may be distended with antibody and, indeed, is among the first places antibody accumulates. In the interphase nucleus the inner nuclear membrane is reinforced on its inner surface by a closely applied finely granular *lamina*. A subset of heterochromatin lies against the inner surface of the lamina, and, in places, penetrates it and reaches to the inner nuclear membrane (Figs. 1–25 and 1–26). This heterochromatin forms a rim around the nucleus, interrupted by nuclear pores (Figs. 1–10 and 1–16 to 1–19). During the first meiotic prophase, chromosomes may be attached to the inner surface of the inner membrane and nucleoli may lie there. Although the nuclear envelope cannot be resolved by light microscopy, its location is often revealed as a definite line representing the sum of the nuclear membranes, nuclear cisterna, and lamina.

Nuclear pore complexes represent interruptions in the nuclear membranes. At a pore complex the inner and outer nuclear membranes appear to fuse and their margins thicken to form an annulus as great as 1,000 Å in outside diameter and 600 Å inside. On surface view it is circular or octagonal in outline. By low-power electron microscopy the pore complex may appear as an aperture in the nuclear membranes with a thickened annulus, closed by a thin diaphragm that often contains a central granule. At high resolution the complex appears to be a granular and filamentous structure with eight regularly spaced granules, each about 100 Å in diameter, lying in the rim of the pore. There are, in fact, two sets of eight granules, one set lying at the outer rim associated with the outer nuclear membrane, the other at the inner rim, associated with the inner nuclear membrane (Fig. 1–25). The central gran-

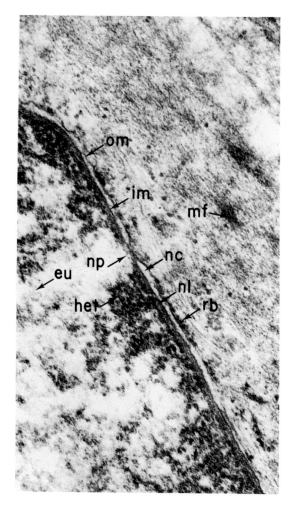

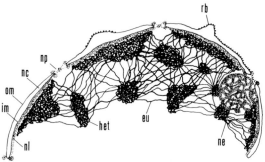

1–25 Above, an electron micrograph of a reticular cell, equine spleen, the nucleus on the left, the cytoplasm on the right. **om** outer nuclear membrane; **im** inner nuclear membrane; **nc** nuclear cisterna; **nl** nuclear lamina; **np** nuclear pore complex; **eu** euchromatin; **het** heterochromatin; **rb** ribosome; **mf** plaque of microfilaments. Courtesy of Fern Tablin. × 42,000. Below, schema of nuclear structures showing, in addition, **ne** nucleolus.

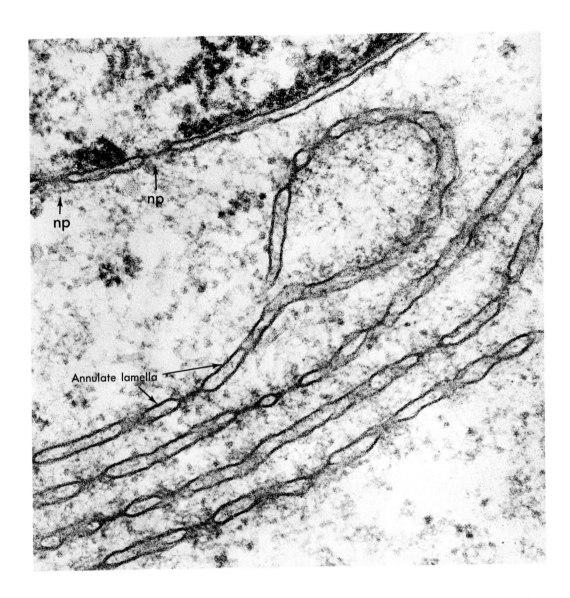

ule is connected by filaments to the wall of the pore complex and to the annular granules. The granules and filaments may be surrounded by a particulate material. The central granule may be traversed by a slender aperture, connecting nucleoplasm with cytoplasm (Fig. 1–19).

There are very few cell types, such as the spermatozoa of bulls, that have few or even no nuclear pore complexes. In other cell types, 3 to 35% of the nuclear surface may be covered by complexes. They may be distributed over the whole nuclear surface or clustered. They may lie irregularly or regularly, falling into square or hexagonal arrays.

Nuclear pore complexes would seem to rep-

1–26 Nuclear pores and annulate lamellae. The nucleus in the left upper corner is bounded by a double membrane, each component consisting of a unit membrane (see text). Within the nucleus, densely stained chromatin is arranged against the nuclear membrane, in which two nuclear pores **(np)** are present. Within the cytoplasm, occupying much of the field, are stacks of annulate lamellae. These appear identical in structure with the nuclear membrane and, like the nuclear membrane, have frequently spaced pore complexes. × 65,000. (From Maul, G. 1970. J. Cell Biol. 46:604.)

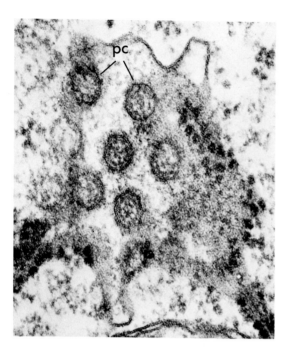

1–27 Annulate lamellae. In this face-on section, surface views of the pore complexes **(pc)** are presented. The pores appear limited by a unit membrane and have a complex, regular internal structure. × 65,000. (From Maul, G. 1970. J. Cell. Biol. 46:604.)

resent passageways, albeit restricted ones, between nucleus and cytoplasm.

Annulate Lamellae. In many cell types stacks of membranes that exactly resemble portions of nuclear membranes, pore complexes and all, may be found in the cytoplasm (Figs. 1–26 and 1–27). In germ cells they may also be present in nucleoplasm. These membranes are termed *annulate lamellae* and are especially common in germ cells and in some tumor cells. They may be continuous with ER. Their significance is not known.

The Cytoplasm

The cytoplasm surrounds the nucleus and is bounded peripherally by the plasma membrane. The cytoplasm expresses most of the functions of the cell. It is dependent on the nucleus for direction, renewal, and regeneration. Thus, isolated units of cytoplasm, exemplified by blood plate-

lets and mature erythrocytes, are capable of protein synthesis and of such specific functions as respiration and the retraction of blood clots. The cytoplasmic structures, however, such as membranes, granules, and microfilaments, which are the basis of such cytoplasmic functions, were originally synthesized and accumulated in the cytoplasm from ribosomes and other materials derived from a viable nucleus that was present at an early phase in the life cycle of these anucleate structures. The volume of cytoplasm in proportion to the nucleus, the nuclear–cytoplasmic ratio, varies considerably from cell type to cell type. In some cells, such as spermatozoa and small lymphocytes, the cytoplasm is scant. In most cells the cytoplasm is relatively abundant and exceeds the nuclear volume by a factor of 3 to 5 or more. The cytoplasm possesses distinctive organelles with specialized functions that lie in the ground substance or hyaloplasm.

Cytoplasm in the center of the cell next to the nucleus, may be gelated. It contains the centrioles and centrosphere but is usually clear of other organelles. It may be bounded by microtubules and surrounded by the Golgi apparatus. Often it pushes the nucleus aside, indenting it. This zone is called the *cell center* or *cytocentrum*. Peripheral to this zone is a solvated part of the cell containing vacuoles and granules, mitochondria, and elements of the ER. Cytoplasmic streaming occurs here, carrying the cytoplasmic organelles in rapid movement. This zone is called *endoplasm*. The peripheral cytoplasm in many cell types, particularly in free or motile cells, is gelated and often rich in microfilaments but free of other organelles. This zone is the *ectoplasm*. It is capable of rapid sol-gel transformation. Gelated ectoplasm may become liquid, particularly in motile cells or cells extending pseudopodial processes, and the already liquid endoplasm bearing organelles then flows in.

The structural protein of the hyaloplasm has a reticulated character visible in high-voltage electron micrographs (Fig. 1–8), which underscores the importance in providing the framework of the cell. Fat occurs in macromolecular micelles that may be visible. Fat sometimes coalesces to form larger fatty vacuoles, *not* bound by membrane, that are visible by electron and light microscopy (Chap. 5). Granules of glycogen may lie in the hyaloplasm, in clusters termed *alpha particles* (Fig. 1–28). However, the predominant structures carried in the hyaloplasm

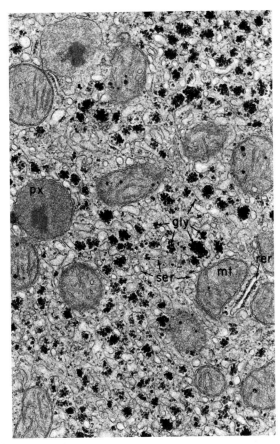

1–28 Glycogen. This electron microscopic field contains particles of glycogen **(gly).** The individual particles are termed beta particles. Ten to fifteen beta particles form an alpha particle. When glycogen is present in lysosomes, presumably to be broken down to glucose and utilized, the glycogen–lysosome structure may be termed *glycosome*. The field also contains peroxisomes **(px),** mitochondria, and endoplasmic reticulum. Most of the endoplasmic reticulum is smooth **(ser)** and contains the glycogen, a finding suggesting that smooth er has a role in glycogen synthesis. × 23,000. (From the work of Robert R. Cardell, Jr.)

are complex organelles fashioned of membranes, filaments, tubules, and granules, which we shall consider now.

Mitochondria. Mitochondria are membranous cytoplasmic organelles capable of trapping chemical energy released by oxidation of compounds derived from food. They then fix that en-

ergy in a form, *adenosine triphosphate (ATP)*, that is readily utilizable by the cell. They are present as punctate or linear structures just within the resolving power of the light microscope (Figs. 1–4 and 1–29). By electron microscopy, mitochondria are tubular or spherical structures bounded by one membrane called the *outer membrane* and containing a second internal folded membrane termed the *inner membrane* (Figs. 1–30 and 1–31).

A cell obtains energy from substrates derived from food. Thus amino acids derived from protein, fatty acids from fat, and glucose from carbohydrate may be sources of energy. The major source, however, is glucose. Glucose is broken down in the cell by glycolytic enzymes to form pyruvic acid, which is then oxidized to acetyl coenzyme A. This compound then proceeds to a cycle of further oxidations, the Krebs tricarboxylic acid cycle, whose end products are carbon dioxide and water. Approximately 690,000 calories of energy per mole lie in the chemical bonds of glucose. Its breakdown to pyruvate yields approximately 40,000 calories per mole, but its complete oxidation to carbon dioxide and water through the Krebs cycle yields another 650,000 calories per mole. The energy-capturing mechanism of cells is at best only about 50% efficient, however, because half of the energy is lost as heat. Therefore, the total caloric content of glucose is never available.

Only about 350,00 calories per mole are useful to the cell. The glycolytic breakdown of glucose is anaerobic—that is, it does not use oxygen. In contrast, the mechanism of the Krebs cycle does require oxygen and is therefore respiratory in nature. The oxidation through the Krebs cycle is of the greatest importance, as indicated by its caloric yields; indeed, it is necessary to life. Blocking this system, as can be done with fluoracetate, causes death. *The Krebs cycle enzymes are present in mitochondria.*

The energy resulting from the oxidation of pyruvate to carbon dioxide and water would, by itself, yield only heat. For this energy to be of value to the metabolism of the cell, it must first be chemically fixed or stored in certain molecules and then be readily released from these molecules as needed. The cell accomplishes this by means of a distinctive enzyme system coupled into the Krebs cycle: the electron-transfer system of cytochromes. This system accepts the energy liberated in each of the steps of the Krebs

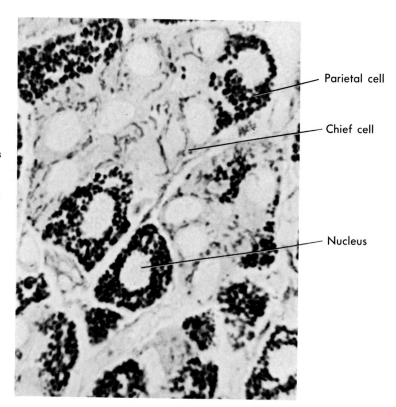

1–29 Light micrograph of a portion of the stomach lining. The preparation has been stained for NAD⁺-dependent isocitric dehydrogenase activity (consult Chap. 2). This constitutes a selective stain for mitochondria. Nuclei are present in negative image. Two cell types are present. One, the parietal cell, is rich in granular mitochondria and carries out active transport. The second, the chief cell, has relatively few filamentous mitochondria and is concerned with the synthesis of protein. These cell types are discussed in Chap. 19. × 1,500. (From the work of D. G. Walker.)

Parietal cell

Chief cell

Nucleus

cycle and incorporates it into so-called high-energy phosphate compounds, notably ATP. This is done by the conversion of *adenosine diphophate (ADP)* to ATP. The additional phosphate bond so formed represents approximately 7,300 calories of stored energy. *The cytochrome electron-transfer system capable of fixing the energy obtained from the oxidations of the Krebs cycle into ATP lies in mitochondria.* The source of energy for virtually every energy-requiring activity of the cell is ATP. It is translocated from mitochondria into surrounding cytoplasm and its energy is released by ATPases, which lie at different locations in the cell. One depot rich in ATPase is the cell membrane. Here the energy obtained from the conversion of ATP to ADP is used in the active transport of compounds across the cell membrane.

Mitochondria may be observed in living cells by phase-contrast microscopy (Fig. 1–1). They are quite pliant and appear to be carried passively in cytoplasmic streams, twisted, bent, and changing shape. On occasion they appear contractile or motile. They are subject to swelling in certain physiological states.

Mitochondria may be vitally stained with Janus green B, pinacyanole, or other vital dyes that exist in either a colored oxidized form or a colorless reduced form. Because of their oxidative enzymes, mitochondria are able to maintain the dye in its oxidized form (a green or blue in the case of Janus green B), whereas the rest of the cytoplasm is usually unable to do so. Mitochondria stand out clearly as stained linear or punctate structures (Figure 11–5).

In fixed and stained light-microscopic preparations, mitochondria are usually demonstrated by virtue of the phospholipid contained in their membranes. Iron hematoxylin is an excellent stain for mitochondria that is used in the Regaud, Baker, and other methods, because it stains phospholipid. Sudan black B or other dyes that dissolve in lipid stain mitochondria faintly.

Mitochondria may also be demonstrated under the light microscope by cytochemical staining of the activity of their enzymes (Fig. 1–29). Thus stains that reveal the activity of succinic dehydrogenase, malic dehydrogenase, isocitrate dehydrogenase, fumaric dehydrogenase, and other oxidative enzymes effectively stain mitochondria. The cells must be carefully fixed to limit diffusion of enzymes and to retain structural clarity. Even slightly prolonged fixation destroys enzyme activity and renders the methods ineffective. Cytochemical methods provide valuable physiological information. For example, mitochondria may appear identical by methods that depend on phospholipid staining or by supravital staining or phase microscopy. Yet in such mitochondria, Krebs-cycle enzymes may have different activity, and by staining for a variety of these enzymes different functional classes of mitochondria may be recognized.

By electron microscopy, mitochondria may be recognized as distinctive tubular or, occasionally, spherical structures made of inner and outer membranes (Figs. 1–30 and 1–31). The outer membrane is unfolded. The inner membrane is folded to form *cristae*, which extend into the center of the mitochondrion. The space enclosed by the inner membrane is the *inner chamber*. It contains a finely granular material, the *matrix*. The space between outer and inner membrane is the *outer chamber*. In most mammalian cells the cristae are plates or shelves that extend partway across the inner chamber. In cardiac muscle and in kidney tubular cells there may be many cristae that reach across the mitochrondrion, whereas in macrophages there are usually few cristae, and they are short. In the testis, ovary, and adrenal gland, the mitochondria of cells secreting steroid hormones have tubular rather than shelflike cristae.

The unit membrane is modified in the cristae. The surface exposed to the inner chamber possesses knoblike repeating units attached to a basal membrane by slender stalks (Fig. 1–32). These units, called *elementary particles*, are best revealed at high magnification with negative staining after osmotic shock. Elementary particles contain a mitochondrial ATPase complex that appears to provide a channel for proton translocation. Normally the particles may be embedded in the membrane rather than project from it.

Mitochondria are subject to conformational change (Figs. 1–30 and 1–31). The *orthodox form*, described above, is typical of mitochondria in tissue section, since the methods of preparation usually result in low levels of ADP with the mitochondria inactive in oxidative phosphorylation. If, however, oxidative phosporylation is induced in isolated mitochondria by adding ADP or if measures are taken to maintain a high level of oxidative phosphorylation in tissue sections, a *condensed mitochrondrial conformation* is revealed. In this form the volume of the outer chamber is increased to approximately 50% of the organelle, and the inner chamber is reduced in volume.

Mitochondria may be isolated relatively easily by a technique that requires disruption of cells and centrifugation of the fragments. In density-gradient centrifugation, the mitochondria form a tan colored stratum lying above the nuclei and below the lysosomes and ribosomes.

Isolated mitochondria exhibit the reactions described above. In addition, they may be studied by standard chemical and microchemical methods. They may be dissociated by applying deoxycholate and other surface-active agents; in this way it has been shown that the electron-transfer system of cytochromes is firmly bound to membranes, whereas the enzymes of the Krebs tricarboxylic acid cycle are not. Electron-microscopic cytochemistry demonstrates the presence of cytochrome oxidase and other oxidative enzymes in sections of mitochondria.

Freeze-fracture-etch methods reveal particles in mitochondrial membranes (Fig. 1–33). The particles on the inner membrane are numerous and may constitute the enzymes of the electron-transfer chain of cytochrome enzymes.

The number and size of mitochondria are, in general, correlated with the level of oxidative phosphorylation. Hepatocytes may each contain about 1,000 to 1,500 mitochondria. Mature erythrocytes, totally dependent for energy on glycolysis, contain none.

Mitochondria may bear characteristic relationships to other organelles and cell structures. Their relationship is often of functional significance, as the mitochondrion is the primary source of energy. Thus in cells synthesizing protein, mitochondria may occur close to ribosomes. In cells engaged in large-scale active transport of materials across a cell membrane, such as the parietal cell of the stomach (which pumps protons across the plasma membrane in the production of hydrochloric acid), the plasma membrane dips into the cell in many folds and mitochondria are closely held in them. In striated muscle cells, which contain myofilaments that slide on one another to effect contraction, mitochondria are present close to the myofilaments. In the development of fat cells, the minute fat droplets that form and then coalesce are intimately associated with mitochondria.

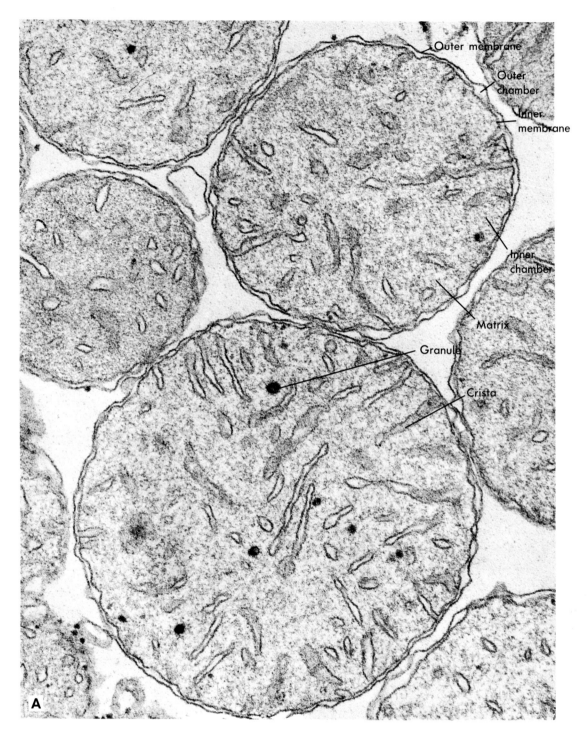

Outer membrane

Outer chamber

Inner membrane

Inner chamber

Matrix

Granule

Crista

A

1–30 Mitochondria of a rat hepatocyte. Mitochondria undergo reversible ultrastructural transformations between a condensed and an orthodox conformation in relationship to the level on oxidative phosphorylation (see text). These changes may be observed in isolated mitochondria and in tissue section. Mitochondria are isolated from disrupted hepatocytes and sectioned. **A.** The conventional

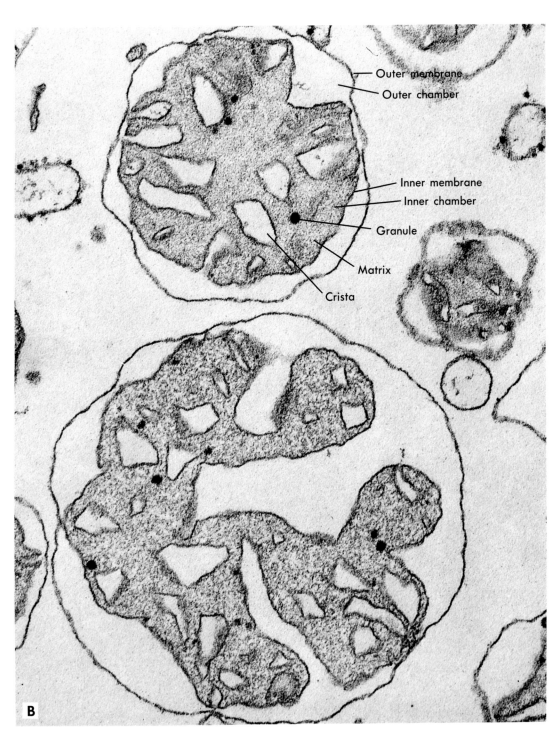

conformation, the outer membrane, outer chamber, inner membrane with cristae, and inner chamber containing matrix and granules may be seen. **B.** The condensed state: the outer chamber is considerably enlarged and the inner membrane and matrix thereby condensed. Each × 110,000. (From Hackenbrock, C. R., 1968. J. Cell Biol. 37:345.)

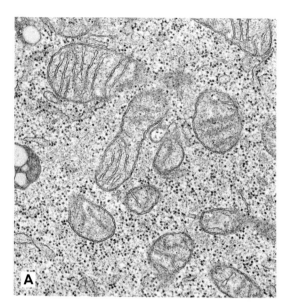

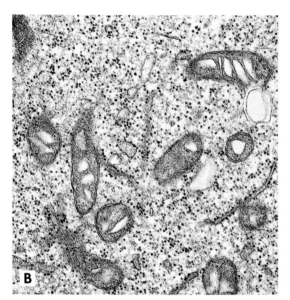

1–31 Mitochondria of an ascites tumor cell. **A.**
△   Mitochondria are present in the orthodox
conformation. A mitochondrion is enclosed in an
outer membrane. The inner membrane is folded into
cristae that extend into the matrix of inner chamber.
× 26,800. **B.** The condensed form, wherein the outer
chamber is expanded, is evident. The cytoplasm also
contains polyribosomes and rough ER. × 26,800.
(From Hackenbrock, C. R., Rehn, T. G., Weinbach,
E. C., and Lemasters, J. J. 1971. J. Cell Biol. 51:123.)

1–32 Mitochondrion from beef heart; negatively
▽   stained electron micrograph. **A.** The cristae of
the mitochondrion are outlined at a magnification of
62,000. Note that small bodies **(arrow)** appear on the
outer cristal membrane facing the interior of the
mitochondrion. **B.** Under 420,000 magnification these
small bodies, the elementary particles **(EP),** are seen
attached to the cristal membrane by a slender
stalk. (From Fernandez-Moran, H., Oda, T., Blair,
P. V., and Green, D. E. 1964. J. Cell Biol. 22:63.)

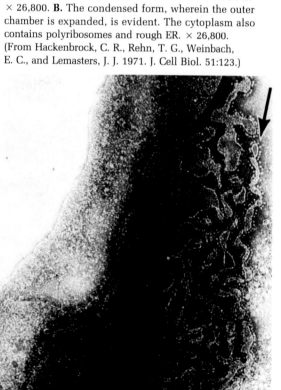

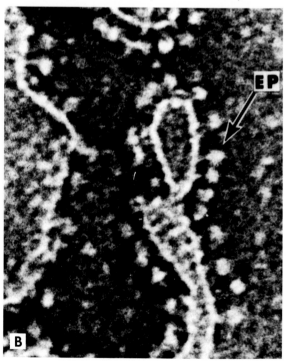

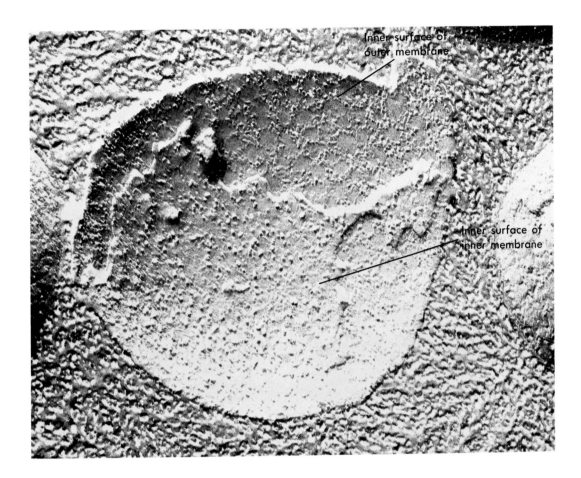

Inner surface of outer membrane

Inner surface of inner membrane

The primary function of mitochondria is respiratory, as has been described. They may display other activities as well, notably the concentration of cations. The dense granules of the mitochondrial matrix in the inner chamber may represent concentrations of Ca^{++}.

Mitochondria contain circular DNA typical of prokaryotes, and mitochondrial ribosomes are similar to bacterial ribosomes in several respects. There is evidence, moreover, that existing mitochondria produce new mitochondria. It is possible that in the evolution of eukaryotes, ancestral prokaryote structures established a felicitous symbiotic relationship and permitted the highly successful evolution of eukaryotes. Alternatively, the prokaryotic character of mitochondrial nucleoproteins may be the result of later eukaryotic evolution (convergent evolution) without any contribution of symbiotic prokaryotic organisms.

Endoplasmic Reticulum. The endoplasmic reticulum (ER) is a cytoplasmic system of tubules,

1–33 Mitochondria of a rat hepatocyte. Freeze-fracture-etch of isolated mitochondria. The fracture line exposed the inner surface of the outer membrane and the inner surface of the inner membrane. Note the rather regularly arranged system of granules on the inner surface of the outer membrane. The granules are the size of certain enzymes and may represent membrane-associated enzymes. × 110,000. (From the work of C. R. Hackenbrock.)

vesicles, and sacs or cisternae fashioned of membranes. It is continuous with the outer membrane of the nuclear envelope (Fig. 1–34). The development of ER varies with cell type and function.

The ER has been defined by electron microscopy, although it has been observed by light microscopy in some cells, notably as the sarcoplasmic reticulum, the specialized ER of striated muscle (Chap. 7). The ER was first described in fibroblasts in tissue culture examined in electron micrographs of whole mounts, i.e., without sec-

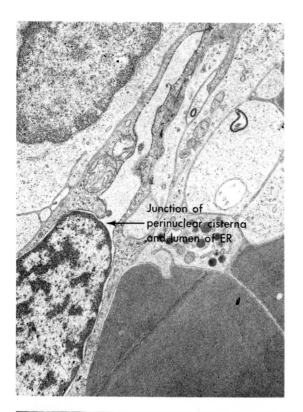

Junction of
perinuclear cisterna
and lumen of ER

1–34 Connective tissue cell from human embryo
spleen. Here the continuity of the outer nuclear
membrane and the smooth ER is evident. Thus the
perinuclear space and the lumen of the ER are
continuous. × 12,000.

◁

1–35 Fibroblast, tissue culture. The preparation in
this electron micrograph has not been
sectioned. It is a whole mount of the cell, and only
the peripheral region is sufficiently thin to permit
passage of the electron beam. (From the work of K. R.
Porter.) ▽

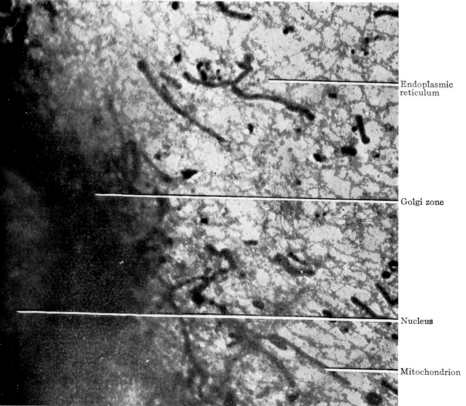

Endoplasmic
reticulum

Golgi zone

Nucleus

Mitochondrion

tioning. Ordinarily, whole cells are too thick for electron-microscopic study, but cells in culture may put out cytoplasmic processes thin enough to pass an electron beam. In such preparations the ER may be seen as a cytoplasmic network (Fig. 1–35).

Two major forms of ER occur. They are *rough* or *granular* ER (Fig. 1–36), which has ribosomes on its outside surface, and *smooth* or *agranular* ER, whose surface is free of ribosomes. Ribosomes synthesize protein (see below) and need not be associated with ER. The association of ER and ribosomes occurs in cells that bind the protein they produce in membranous sacs. For example, erythroblasts synthesize the protein hemoglobin, which remains dispersed through the cytoplasm; thus, ribosomes are plentiful but little ER is present. In plasma cells, on the other hand, which synthesize large volumes of antibody, confine it by membranes, and then secrete it, rough ER is abundant. Peptide chains are synthesized in the ribosomes and sent across the ER membrane into the lumen of the ER. The ER thereby isolates synthesized material from the rest of the cytoplasm, permits further assembly of peptides into larger molecules, and conveys the material by means of *transport vesicles* to the Golgi complex where further synthesis and processing occur. The Golgi then release the secretion enclosed in membranous sacs, the *condensing vacuoles*, which mature into secretory vacuoles. (See discussion of the Golgi complex, page 48.) Rough ER, well developed in secretory cells, is also abundant in cells that synthesize protein and hold it membrane-bounded within their cytoplasm, as in leukocytes and macrophages. These cells contain enzyme-rich membrane-bounded granules, the *lysosomes*. The formation of these granules parallels the formation of secretory vacuoles, except that the granules tend to be retained rather than released (secreted). The process of secretion is fully discussed in Chap. 21. See, particularly, Figs. 21–9 to 21–13.

In nerve cells rough ER exists as large, flattened sacs lying on one another in lamellated fashion to form masses, *Nissl bodies*, identifiable by light microscopy. Hepatic parenchymal

1–36 Hepatocyte of a rat. In this portion of the cytoplasm most of the cisternae of the rough ER were cut transversely and others tangentially. In the latter **(arrow)** the membrane of the ER and the attached polysomes are seen *en face*. A section of a mitochondrion **(mit)** is present. × 64,000. (From the work of G. E. Palade.)

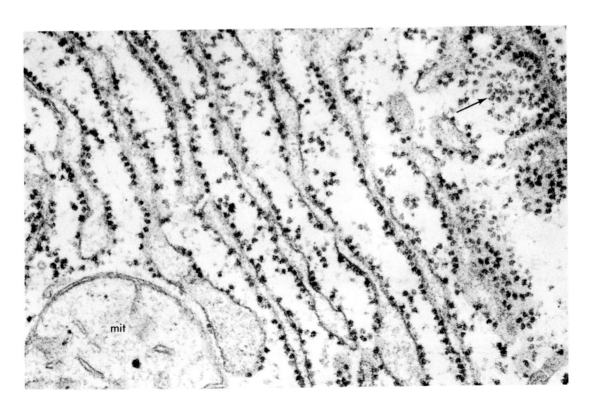

mit

cells contain smaller blocks of rough ER. In plasma cells the rough ER is rather uniformly distributed through the cytoplasm except in the region of the cytocentrum. It may be tubular, vesicular, or flattened, depending on the phase of antibody secretion. Rough ER occupies the base of the pancreatic acinar cell. This rough ER, recognizable by light microscopy as basophilic material (because of the affinity of its ribosomes for cationic dye) is termed *ergastoplasm* (Figs. 1–3 and 1–4).

Smooth ER, free of ribosomes, occurs in a number of cell types and may have diverse functions. It has a role in the production of steroid hormones and it is abundant in such cells as the Leydig cells of the testis, which produce the steroid testosterone. Smooth ER synthesizes complex lipids from fatty acids. It also detoxifies certain drugs and becomes very prominent in hepatocytes during the inactivation of phenobarbital. In striated muscle, smooth ER is distinctly organized as the sarcoplasmic reticulum whose functions include delivering high concentrations of Ca^{++} and other ions to critical places in the sarcomere for muscular contraction and relaxation. Smooth ER in megakaryocytes delimits platelet zones in the cytoplasm and, by fusing, frees platelets from the megakaryocyte. Appropriately, this ER is termed "demarcation membrane". Carbohydrate synthesis is associated with smooth ER and the Golgi apparatus. The reformation of the nuclear membrane in telophase is accomplished by smooth ER.

The membranes of the ER possess a self-healing capacity after disruption. When fractions rich in ER are recovered from disrupted ultracentrifuged cells, the ER is found as small vesicles *(microsomes)* (Fig. 1–37). Evidently the tubular system is fragmented, but the membranes reunite or "heal" to form small vesicles. After fixation with osmium tetroxide (but not gluteraldehyde) the tubular T system of sarcoplasmic reticulum is revealed as an artifactual system of vesicles— another example of the readiness with which the tubules of ER may be broken up and reformed as small vesicles.

Ribosomes. A single ribosome is below the limit of resolution of the light microscope, but in aggregate, the presence of ribosomes can be recognized. Owing, in all likelihood, to their PO_4^{3-} groups, they have a pronounced affinity for cationic or basic dyes such as methylene blue$^+$. As a result, cells rich in ribosomes are basophilic;

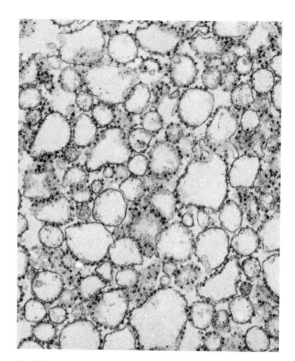

1–37 Microsomes of rat liver. The liver was disrupted and various fractions recovered by ultracentrifugation. This is the microsome fraction. It consists almost entirely of rough ER that had been disrupted and "healed" as vesicles. Ribosomes remain attached to the outer surface. × 40,000. (From the work of D. Sabatini and M. Adelman.)

this basophilia may be abolished by pretreating the tissue with ribonuclease. The intensity and disposition of the basophilia are highly characteristic of cell type. Basophilic material visualized by light microscopy has been designated *chromidial substance*. Consult the description of pancreatic islet cells (Chap. 22), lymphocytes (Chap. 11), and erythroblasts (Chap. 12) for patterns of chromidial substance.

Ribosomes are flattened, spheroidal, complex cytoplasmic particles measuring approximately 150 × 250 Å that synthesize protein (Figs. 1–38 to 1–41). They consist of RNA and protein. Their RNA is classed as rRNA, which accounts for 85% of the RNA of the cell. In addition to this form of RNA, there is mRNA and tRNA. The instruction for protein synthesis is encoded in DNA. This information is transcribed to mRNA, which is about 300 to 600 nm long, depending on the protein. Messenger RNA is produced in the nucleus, on a template of uncoiled DNA. It moves to the

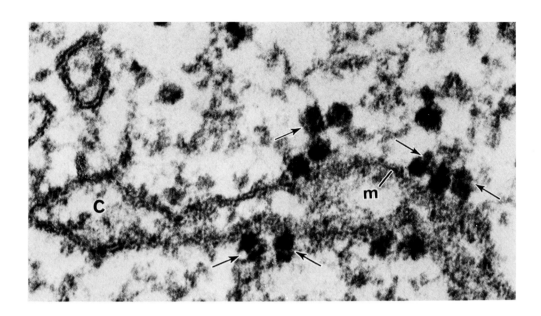

cytoplasm where it associates itself with ribosomes that lie along the mRNA like beads on a necklace. Ribosomes occurring singly in the cytoplasm are not active; only when they are linked by mRNA to form polyribosomes do they engage in protein synthesis. The ribosomes are the small machines that receive the amino acid constituents of protein, assemble them into peptide chains, and release these chains into the cytoplasm or into the lumen of the ER where they continue to aggregate to form protein. Each amino acid is brought to the ribosome by its distinctive tRNA, a low molecular-weight nucleic acid (see below) that may be produced in the nucleolar region of the nucleus (as is rRNA) and passes out of the nucleus into the cytoplasm. In protein synthesis, a ribosome moves along mRNA and reads the genetic message that has been transcribed from DNA. As the ribosome translates the message, it binds on its surface the particular activated amino acyl-tRNA specified by the codon being read and synthesizes the peptide linkage of this amino acid to the earlier ones.

The peptide chain grows larger as the ribosome moves along the mRNA, and as the ribosomes slides off the mRNA, it releases the peptide chain. As one ribosome slides off one end of the mRNA, another slides onto the other end and several ribosomes "read" or translate the mRNA at any time. The ribosomes lie on the mRNA approximately 340 Å apart (Fig. 1–40). For a poly-

1–38 Ribosomes, hepatocyte, of a guinea pig.

Ribosomes at high magnification show a larger and smaller component. When associated with the ER, the larger component lies upon the membrane. In this field a single cisterna (c) of the ER is present. The arrows indicate the position and orientation of the partitions separating the large from the small subunits of the ribosomes. Note that these partitions lie generally parallel to the surface of the membranes (m). This specimen was fixed in osmium tetroxide, embedded, sectioned, and stained with uranyl acetate. × 270,000. (From the work of D. Sabatini, Y. Toshiro, and G. E. Palade.)

peptide chain of hemoglobin 150 amino acids long, 60 to 90 sec are required for the ribosome to run the length of mRNA.

The ribosome is composed of two unequal subunits, one large and the other small (Fig. 1–42). Both are highly organized macromolecular assemblies consisting of one or more RNA molecules and numerous different proteins. In humans, as in most eukaryotes, the smaller subunit has a molecular weight of 1.5×10^6 and is composed of a single molecule of RNA with a sedimentation constant of 18S and approximately 30 different, rather small proteins (10,000 to 40,000 daltons). The small subunit functions to bind the mRNA to the ribosome and forms part of the tRNA binding site as the codon is being read by the anticodon of the tRNA. The larger subunit with a molecular weight of 3.0 ×

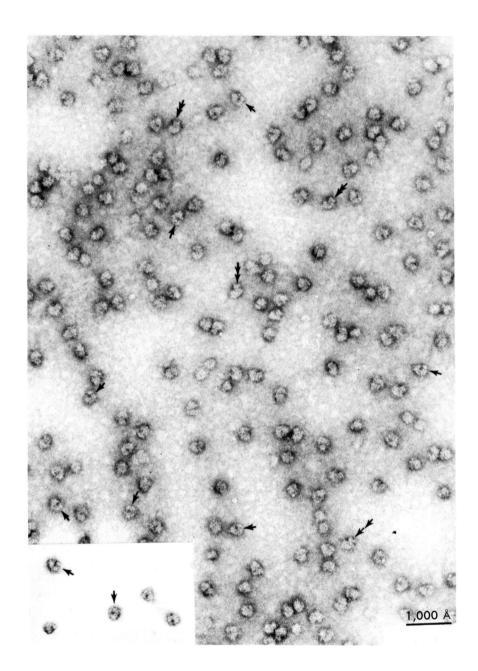

1–39 Ribosomes of a guinea pig. General view of a
field of native monomeric ribosomes. Several
image types are predominant. Frontal images **(arrows)**
have an elongated small subunit profile and a dense
spot toward the side of the separation between
subunits. All frontal images in the field have this spot
to the left of the observer if the particle image is
oriented with the elongated small subunit horizontally
and toward the top. In lateral images **(double arrows)**
the small subunit produces a small rounded or
rectangular profile toward one side of the large
subunit profile. The inset shows images of
monomeric ribosomes, reconstituted in vitro from the
isolated large and small subunits. This preparation
was made from ribosomes isolated by differential
centrifugation of disrupted cells. The ribosomes were
then floated on a membrane-covered electron-
microscopic grid, dried, and negatively stained with
phosphotungstic acid. × 125,000. (From the work of
D. Sabatini, Y. Nonomura, and G. Blobel.)

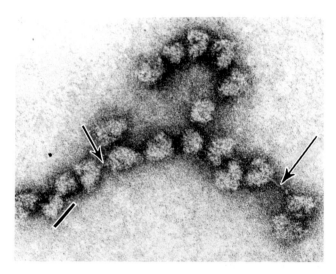

1–40 Ribosomes of a guinea pig. Here a strand of messenger RNA **(arrows)** links ribosomes into a polyribosomal unit. The mRNA runs between the small and large subunits. × 240,000. (From the work of D. Sabatini, Y. Nonomura, and G. Blobel.)

◁

1–41 An electron micrograph of *E. coli* small ribosomal subunits reacted with antibodies directed against ribosomal protein S14. The antibodies attach at only a single region in the upper one-third of the subunit, and are indicated by arrows. The centrally located pairs of subunits are connected by single IgG molecules, while the pair of subunits on the left is connected by two different IgG molecules, both attached to the same region of the subunit surface. (From the work of J. Lake, M. Pendergast, L. Kahan, and M. Nomura.)

◁

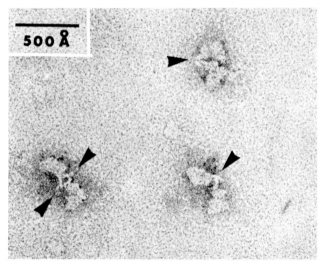

1–42 Model of the *E. coli* ribosome showing the relationship of the large and the small subunits. The view on the left shows the interface between the small subunit **(light)** and the large subunit **(dark).** This interface is an important region where the tRNAs, the mRNA, and factors involved in protein synthesis are located. In the view at the right showing the ribosome viewed from above, a prominent feature of the large subunit is the elongated projection extending from the subunit. At present, the function of this feature of the large subunit is not well understood. (From the work of J. Lake.) ▽

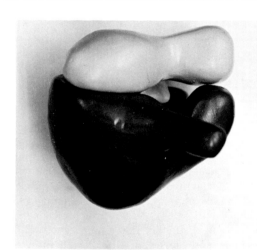

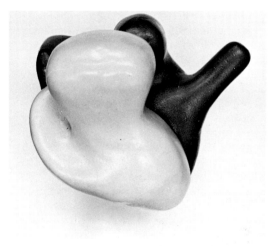

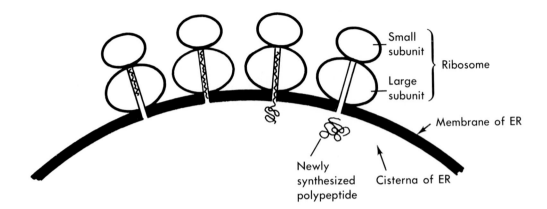

1–43 Model of the relationship between ribosomes and ER membrane. Attachment by the large subunits and orientation of the partition separating the two ribosomal subunits are strongly suggested by the evidence presented. The central channel in the large subunit and the discontinuity in the subjacent ER membrane are tentative features of the model, included only to indicate a possible pathway for the release of the newly synthesized protein in the cisternal space. (From the work of D. Sabatini and G. Blobel.)

10^6 has a sedimentation constant of 60S and contains two RNA molecules (5S and 28S) and probably a third (5.8S). The approximately 40 different proteins contained in the large subunit are on the average slightly larger than those in the small subunit. The large subunit functions in protein synthesis by forming part of the tRNA binding sites, catalyzing peptidyl transfer, and holding the growing polypeptide chain. Ribosomes bound to the rough ER are attached through the large subunit (Fig. 1–43). In bacteria, and prokaryotes in general, ribosomes (70S) and their subunits (30S and 50S) are somewhat smaller. Bacterial ribosomes differ from eukaryotic ribosomes in their responses to antibiotics affecting protein synthesis. Some antibiotics, such as puromycin, inhibit protein synthesis on both prokaryotic and eukaryotic ribosomes; others, such as cycloheximide, affect only eukaryotic ribosomes. (The ribosomes found in the mitochondria of eukaryotes differ from others in eukaryotic cytoplasm by resembling bacterial ribosomes in their responses to antibiotics.) Eukaryotic and prokaryotic ribosomes have important similarities despite their differences. The sequence of events that occur during the protein synthesis cycle is the same in both eukaryotic and prokaryotic ribosomes, and although there are differences in size, these ribosomes greatly resemble each other in gross morphology as observed in the electron microscope.

The three-dimensional locations of specific ribosomal proteins are being mapped by using antibodies directed against individual ribosomal proteins (Figs. 1–41 and 1–44).

Polyribosomes may lie free in the cytoplasm, releasing their peptide chains into the cytoplasm for further combination and complexing. This is how hemoglobin is synthesized. Where the ribosomes attach to the outer surface of ER, the larger unit maintains attachment. The mRNA and the ER membranes are parallel. Furthermore, there may be a canal running through the larger ribosomal component at right angles to the mRNA and the ER. This canal has been postulated to run through the membranous wall of the ER, with the result that the amino acids, in peptide linkage, are "spun out" by the ribosomes directly into the lumen of the ER (Fig. 1–43). This peptide is "led" across the wall of the ER into its lumen by a signal peptide produced by the large ribosomal subunit and linked to the amino terminal of the peptide. See Chap. 21 for further discussion of secretion.

Ribosomes have a short life span. When protein synthesis ceases, they are quickly metabolized and disappear.

Golgi Complex. The Golgi apparatus or complex is a membranous system of cisternae and vesicles, usually located in or around the cytocentrum. It is involved in intracellular transport of secretory proteins, membrane proteins, and proteins that remain membrane-bounded within the cell, in distinction to proteins such as hemoglobin and keratin that lie free in the cytoplasm.

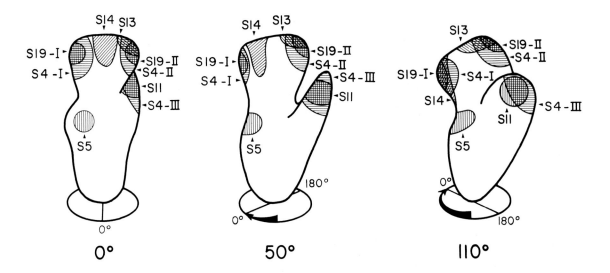

1-44 A diagrammatic representation of three views of the E. coli smaller ribosomal subunit illustrating the locations of some of the ribosomal proteins. The views from left to right represent rotations of the subunit about its long axis of 0°, 50°, and 110°, respectively. The cleft formed between the vertically oriented platform and the upper one-third of the subunit is best seen in the +50° view. The platform itself is attached to the lower two-thirds of the subunit. The vertical axis of the subunit is approximately 250 Å long. Many of the proteins are located at only a single region of the subunit but some, such as S4 and S19, are elongated and extend through the subunit. Three different regions of S4 are exposed and indicate that this protein must be at least 170 Å long. Protein S4 is required for the proper self-assembly of subunits and its extended nature may be related to its role in subunit assembly. (From the work of J. Lake, M. Nomura, and L. Kahan.)

The Golgi complex has a characteristic appearance by light microscopy. It may be a small compact structure; it may be a cluster of small structures (termed dictyosomes in earlier literature); or it may be a large netlike structure, the *internal reticular apparatus* as initially defined by C. Golgi in nerve cells. The Golgi complex is often juxtanuclear and may partially enclose the centrioles. Its size fluctuates with cell type and secretory activity. It is well developed in secretory cells, for example, in the mucus-producing intestinal epithelial cells, in plasma cells, and cells of the pituitary gland. The Golgi complex has the capacity to reduce metal salts, such as salts of osmium and of silver (Figs. 1–4 and 1–45), and may therefore be stained with these compounds. Such staining methods were responsible for the discovery of the Golgi complex.

By electron microscopy, the Golgi complex consists of 3 to 15 large flat sacs or cisternae apposed to one another. They are relatively compressed at their centers and somewhat dilated peripherally. The sacs tend to be bowed, presenting a convex *proximal face* (toward the nucleus) and concave *distal face* (away from the nucleus (Figs 1–35 to 1–37, 21–9, and 22–8). These stacked cisternae thus form bowl-shaped structures, and the Golgi complex as a whole looks like a stack of shallow bowls with the concavity directed away from the nucleus. The cisternae may communicate with one another by slender channels at places along their contiguous surfaces. The proximal membranes (those near the nucleus) are thinner than the distal membranes (facing out toward the bulk of the cytoplasm), which are more like those of plasmalemma. At the edge of the lamellated sacs, near their expanded peripheries, vesicles 400 to 800 Å in diameter are typically present. Similar vesicles may also be abundant at the distal face. The vesicles vary in size and probably fuse to form larger vesicles. They, like the lateral vesicles, may contain a dense material. The proximal face is relatively free of vesicles and has been termed the *forming face* (also known as the *cis* face). The distal face, which is typically engaged in granule formation, has been termed the *maturation face* (also known as the *trans* face) (Figs. 1–46 to 1–49).

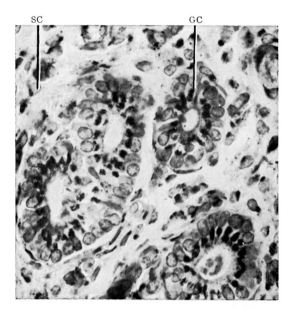

1–45 Golgi material in cells of guinea pig uterus.
     The Golgi material was blackened with silver by the method of Da Fano. Large quantities of it lie above the nuclei of the glandular cells **(GC);** smaller amounts lie next to the nuclei of the stromal cells **(SC).** × 500.

◁

1–46 Human myelocyte. In this developing blood cell (see Chap. 11), the nucleus is lobed. Nuclear pores **(np)** are present. The cytoplasm contains granules, vesicles, rough and smooth ER, mitochondria, and free ribosomes. A Golgi apparatus is present, partially surrounding a centriole. × 26,000. (From the work of G. A. Ackerman.)   ▽

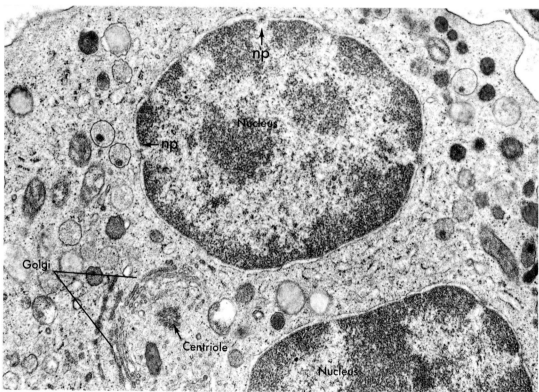

Proteins destined to be secreted or stored in lysosomes or other membrane-bounded granules are synthesized by polysomes attached to the outer surface of ER. Newly synthesized proteins collect within the lumen of the rough ER and move into contiguous ER free of ribosomes.

These elements are called "transitional elements" because they lie between the rough ER and the Golgi complex. It is thought that they bud off as *transport vesicles*, which carry quanta of ER content to the Golgi complex. The Golgi complex not only serves as a way station for pro-

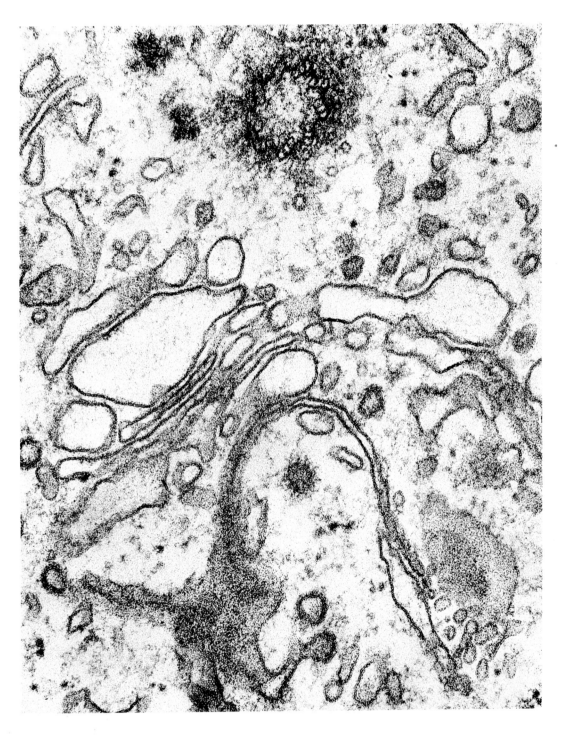

tein intracellular transport, but several covalent modifications of proteins may occur as they pass through it. For example, a portion of the carbohydrate moiety of many glycoproteins is added in the Golgi complex (e.g., immunoglobulins and pancreatic enzymes). The high concentration of

1–47 Golgi complex. It is evident, in this field, that the Golgi membranes and vesicles are made of the trilaminar unit membrane. A centriole is also present. (From the work of E. D. Hay and J. P. Revel.)

the *glycosyl transferase* enzymes on the inner surface of Golgi membranes reflects this function.

There are several patterns of secretion. In "nonregulated" secretory cells (e.g., plasma cells and fibroblasts), secretion is continuous and is effected by small Golgi-derived secretory vesicles, perhaps 50 nm in diameter. In "regulated" secretory cells (e.g., pancreatic acinar cells), on the other hand, secretion is intermittent and depends on hormonal stimuli. In this case, the secretory granules accumulate in the apical cytoplasm and may become rather large, up to 1,500 nm in diameter. In such cells, the ability of the Golgi complex to concentrate secretory protein is especially evident. Distal to the stacked cisternae are "condensing vacuoles" of irregular shape. These organelles further concentrate their content to become zymogen or storage granules. Upon hormonally triggered secretion, the granule membrane fuses with the plasma membrane. At the site of fusion the membranes break down and the contents of the secretory granule are released from the cell. See Figs. 21–9, 21–12, 21–13, and 22–8.

The Golgi complex also functions in lipoprotein synthesis. Lipids enter the Golgi cisternae from smooth ER and in the Golgi apparatus they are complexed to protein produced in rough ER. Membrane-bounded lipoprotein granules are then released from the Golgi (Figs. 1–48 and 1–49).

A major technique for delineating the sequence of protein intracellular transport is *pulse-chase electron-microscopic autoradiography*. With this method, a radioactive metabolite, such as an amino acid or sugar that will be incorporated into the macromolecular product undergoing synthesis, is injected rapidly in a single dose into an experimental animal. As a result, a short, sharply delineated "pulse" of radioactively labeled metabolite enters the synthetic process and is carried through it. By sampling tissue at appropriate times for autoradiography, the "pulse labeled" radioactive macromolecules (e.g., proteins) can be visualized at their site of synthesis and followed during transport to the site of discharge.

The Golgi complex has been isolated by differential centrifugation and has been partially characterized chemically. It consists of approximately equal parts of lipid and protein and tends to be unusually rich in nucleoside diphosphatases. These phosphatases serve as cytochemical

and biochemical markers for Golgi membranes. After a short time an identical but now radioactive compound is digested rapidly. This "chases" the radioactive amino acid, diluting it out.

Smooth Vesicles and Coated Vesicles. The cytoplasm contains several kinds of membrane-bounded vesicles that enclose diverse materials and carry them from place to place within the cytoplasm and to and from the cell surfaces. These vesicles include phagosomes, macropinosomes, micropinosomes, condensing vesicles, transport vesicles and secretory vesicles. Lysosomes, peroxisomes, and microbodies may also be included and are discussed in the next section. The movement and destination of vesicles within the cell may be rather specific. For example, vesicles originating at the cell surface may selectively take in immunoglobulin, transport it across the cell using well-defined cytoplasmic streams, and release it at the lateral or basal surfaces of the cell. In addition, protein, partially synthesized in the ER, may be delivered for further synthesis to the Golgi complex by a system of transport vesicles that bud off the ER, travel to the Golgi sacs, and fuse with them.

The cytoplasm of virtually every cell contains membrane-bounded vesicles originating at the cell surface from invaginations of plasma membrane that pinch off. Because such vesicles carry material from outside into the cell, the process that results in their formation has been called *endocytosis*. In the reverse process, *exocytosis*, intracellular material is conveyed within vesicles to the cell surface where the membrane of the vesicle fuses with the plasma membrane and then breaks down, releasing the material to the extracellular compartment. In the process, the vesicle disappears and its membrane is translocated into the plasma membrane.

In endocytosis, the endocytotic vesicles may contain particulate material, such as bacteria or cell fragments. These vesicles are called *phagocytic* vesicles or *phagosomes*. Phagosomes typically flow toward lysosomes and fuse with them, forming *phagolysosomes, heterolysosomes,* or *secondary lysosomes* (Chap. 4). The hydrolytic enzymes of the lysosomes mix and digest the particulate material of the phagosome, and the resulting low molecular-weight compounds diffuse from the phagolysome into the hyaloplasm. Phagocytic vesicles tend to be large, visible by light microscopy. Certain cell types such as macrophages (Chap. 4) and leukocytes (Chap. 11) are

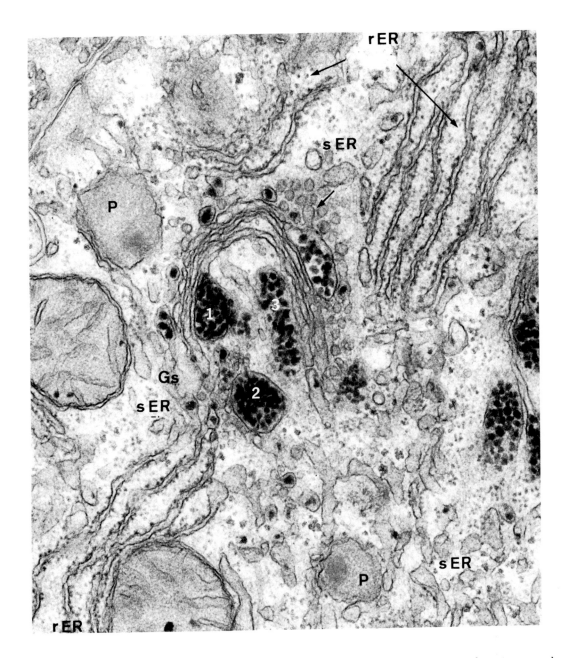

1–48 Golgi complex from a rat hepatocyte. The complex lies near the center of this field. The forming face of the Golgi, where the development of secretory product is initiated, is at the convex side of the apparatus, with extensions from the smooth ER network **(sER)** piling up from below and above, along the curved structure. This smooth ER is probably produced by the rough ER **(rER)** that surrounds the Golgi. The smooth ER may be continuous with the Golgi saccules or may break up into transport vesicles that move to the Golgi and fuse with it. A cluster of small vesicles, on top of the Golgi structure and next to a concentrating or secretory vesicle, is interpreted as representing cross sections of tubular, smooth ER extensions, with one of them **(arrow)** connecting with the concentrating vesicle. At the concave or maturing face of the Golgi three concentrating or secretory vesicles (1 to 3) are present. Each contains many small granules. At P, there are two peroxisomes (see text). Compare this process of lipoprotein granule formation with that of the formation of granules within leukocytes, described in Chap. 11. × 56,500. (From Claude, A. 1970. J. Cell Biol. 47:745.)

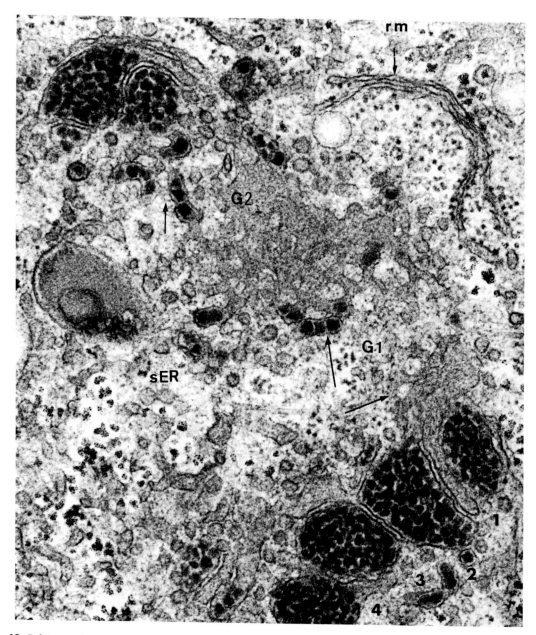

1–49 Golgi complex from a rat hepatocyte. Smooth-surfaced membranes **(rm)** similar to those in Fig. 1–48 are cut in cross section. As they are traced to the right, they are continuous with rough ER. At G2 Golgi membranes at the forming surface are cut in a plane parallel to their surface. These membranes are fenestrated and, in all probability, are formed by coalescence of smooth ER **(sER)** tubules **(arrows)** carrying rows of dense lipoprotein granules. Four large concentrating or secretory vesicles are present (numbered 1 to 4). These would develop from the maturing face of the Golgi, corresponding to the concave portion in Fig. 1–48. × 67,800. (From Claude, A. 1970. J. Cell Biol. 47:745.)

quite proficient or "professional" phagocytes. Other cell types, however, can be phagocytic, such as the endothelium of the vascular sinuses of bone marrow and spleen (Chap. 13), and phagocytosis must be regarded as a general property of cells.

Another class of endocytotic vesicles may contain fluids imbibed from the extracellular fluid at the cell surface. These are *pinocytotic vesicles* or *pinosomes* (*pino*, drinking). Pinosomes may bring fluid in unselectively or they may depend on receptors to bring material into the cell selectively, which is called *receptor mediated pinocytosis*. A type of pinosome is greater than 0.2 μm in diameter. This type is large enough to be visible by light microscopy, and in fact, was first described more than 50 years ago in living cells in tissue culture. These *macropinosomes* characteristically move in cytoplasmic streams toward the center of the cell, becoming smaller and denser as they travel, their contents presumably becoming more concentrated owing to loss of water. Macropinosomes, like phagosomes, may fuse with lysosomes.

A variety of pinocytosis undertaken by virtually every cell of the body, *micropinocytosis*, is distinguished by vesicles visible only by electron microscopy (70 to 100 nm in diameter).

The endocytic vesicular systems function to bring material into a cell, to segregate that material, and to transport it to selective destinations within the cell. In endothelium, for example, vesicles originate at the luminal surface, cross the cell and release their contents at the basal surface. Vesicles may also move in the opposite direction. This type of transit, *transcytosis*, is discussed more fully in Chap. 9. In the epithelial cells lining the gut, materials are taken up at the luminal or apical surface and transported to the lateral cell surface by vesicles and discharged into the intercellular space (Chap. 19). In addition to the discharge of immunoglobulin, the many instances of secretion are examples of exocytosis. Secretory vesicles typically derive from the Golgi complex as *condensing* or *storage vesicles*, and become secretory vesicles, which collect in the apical or secretory pole of the cell. They then move to the cell surface, fuse with the plasma membrane, open to the extracellular space, and discharge their secretion (Figs. 21–9, 21–12, 21–13, and 22–8). Secretion is discussed throughout this book, but major presentations are in the chapters on epithelium (Chap. 3), salivary glands (Chap. 7), mammary glands (Chap. 26), pancreas (Chaps. 21 and 22), and hypophysis

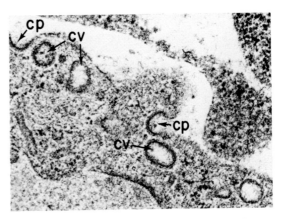

1–50 Endothelium, mouse bone marrow. Coated pits **(cp)** and coated vesicles **(cv)** are present. × 25,000. See also Figs. 3–15, and 8–36.

(Chap. 29), as well as in the earlier sections of this chapter on the endoplasmic reticulum (page 41) and the Golgi complex (page 49).

Cytoplasmic vesicles can be smooth or coated. Smooth vesicles are bounded by membrane similar to the plasma membrane. Coated vesicles are coated on their outside (cytoplasmic) surface by a protein, *clathrin*, of molecular weight 180,000. Clathrin invests the vesicle and appears in sections as radiating spikes, each about 15 nm long and about 5 nm apart, which gives the vesicle a fuzzy look. On surface view the clathrin forms a lattice of hexagons, the side of the polygons being the projections or spikes seen in sections. Coated pinosomes originate as invaginations from coated invaginations of the cell surface, *coated pits* (Figs. 1–50 and 1–51).

Coated and smooth vesicles have similar and complementary functions. Any type of vesicle may be smooth, but coated vesicles are almost always of small diameter (70–10 nm) and only in a few instances are larger. The nature and special functions of coated vesicles are being sorted out. Coated endocytotic vesicles transport immunoglobulin across the placenta from mother to fetus, thereby conferring passive immunity on the fetus. Coated vesicles also transport yolk proteins into the cytoplasm of oocytes. As the yolk-containing coated vesicles move centrally, they lose their clathrin coat and fuse with other yolk-containing vesicles to form rather large yolk vesicles. They, in turn, fuse with lysosomes, and the yolk is digested into low molecular-weight nutrients that diffuse out of the lysosome-yolk vesicle to be metabolized by the oocyte. Casein, as noted above, is carried in exocytotic coated ves-

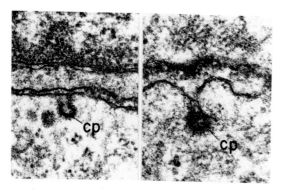

1–51 Leukocytes, mouse bone marrow. Varieties of coated pit **(cp).** left panel × 42,000, right × 70,000. See also Figs. 3–15 and 8–36. Courtesy Joyce S. Knoll

icles that may be rather large. The liver produces a very low density lipoprotein (VLDL) which it releases to the blood through exocytotic coated vesicles. VLDL is a component of blood serum that controls the dispersment of serum lipids, a factor important in the development of atherosclerosis in the walls of the blood vessels. The clathrin coat may play a distinctive role in recycling exocytic membrane. In the synaptic bulb at the end of certain nerves, a number of synaptic vesicles are present. These vesicles are bounded by smooth membrane and contain neurotransmitter substances. When the nerve is stimulated the synaptic vesicles move to the plasma membrane at the synapse, fuse with it, and discharge their contents. After discharge, the membrane of the synaptic vesicle is intercalated into the plasma membrane. It appears that this intercalated membrane may be translocated a short distance away from the synapse and then recycled into the cell where it again forms synaptic vesicles. Clathrin seems to play an essential role in this recycling by moving beneath the translocated synaptic membrane intercalated in the plasma membrane and inducing it to invaginate and pinch off in the cytoplasm as a coated vesicle. When the clathrin first moves beneath the plasma membrane, its latticework is entirely hexagonal. Then pentagons appear in the lattice, and with this change the clathrin assumes a curvilinear form, bringing in the membrane as an invaginated coated pit that proceeds to form a coated vesicle. The coated vesicle next loses its clathrin coat and becomes, once again, a smooth synaptic vesicle. Its clathrin coat appears to prevent a coated vesicle from fusing with other membranous structures. When material is endocytized by a coated vesicle, therefore, that mate-

rial remains within that vesicle as long as it remains coated. When the coat drops away, the membrane of the vesicle may fuse with similar vesicles forming larger vesicles, with lysosomes forming heterolysosomes, with plasma membrane resulting in exocytosis, or with such other membranous structures as the Golgi complex to facilitate transport and synthesis.

Lysosomes, Peroxisomes and Multivesicular Bodies. Lysosomes are membrane-bounded cytoplasmic vesicles containing 50 or more hydrolytic enzymes, virtually all of which are glycoproteins active at acid pH (Figs. 1–52 and 1–53). Lysosomes may become quite large but in their primary state usually measure 50 to 80 Å in diameter. They may be isolated by differential centrifugation of disrupted cells, where they lie centripetal to mitochondria. They may be identified

1–52 Lysosomes of the epithelioid cell of chicken. In this cell, derived from a macrophage, the cytoplasm is filled with lysosomes. They crowd out the centrosome. From the centriole, rays of gelated cytoplasm free of organelles radiate. At one place a small pocket of Golgi membranes is present. (From Sutton, J., and Weiss, L. 1966. J. Cell Biol. 28:303.)

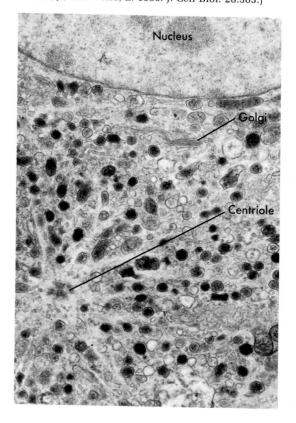

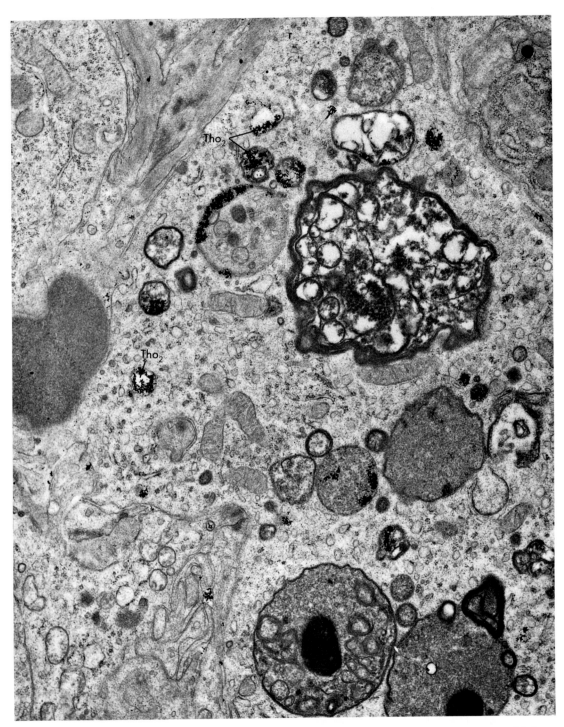

1–53 Lysosomes of a macrophage from a rabbit. This animal was given thorium dioxide (ThO₂), an electron-dense heavy metal, shortly before this cell was fixed. Heterolysosomes, considerably different in appearance, are present. Many contain some ThO₂. × 40,000. (From Weiss, L. 1964. Bull. Hopkins Hosp. 115:99.)

Table 1–3 Major Enzymatic Activities
of Lysosomes

Acid phosphatase
lipase and esterase
phospholipases
ribo- and deoxyribo-nucleases
galactos- and glucos-aminidases
fuco- and gluco-sidases
glucuronidase and hyaluronidase
aryl- and chondro-sulfatases
cathepsins and other peptidases

cytochemically by reactions for acid phosphatase, a commonly used marker, or by reactions for other enzymes they contain. In such cytochemical preparations lysosomes appear as punctate structures by light microscopy. In electron micrographs they are oval or round and contain variably dense granular material. Most cells contain lysosomes. Hepatocytes and macrophages, cell types rich in lysosomes, contain approximately 200. Their large complement of hydrolytic enzymes (Table 1–3) endows lysosomes with the capacity to hydrolyze or digest a great many substrates. The activity of these enzymes is controlled by their bounding membrane. This membrane selectively admits substrates into the lysosome and protects the cells against indiscriminate digestion by its own lysosomal enzymes.

The digestive capacities of lysosomes have been adapted to the functions of disparate cell types. In phagocytic cells, for example, lysosomes digest microbes or other phagosomal contents brought into the cell (heterophagy). In almost any cell of the body, moreover, organelles that have become worn out or exhausted and need to be replaced may be incorporated into lysosomes and digested (autophagy). Furthermore, secretory substances synthesized by endocrine cells may be digested by lysosomal enzymes and the level of secretion thereby regulated (crinophagy). In fact, lysosomes may participate in the destruction and recycling of many cell components, such as receptors and membrane.

The life cycle of lysosomes is complex and accounts for their marked structural heterogeneity (polymorphism). The primary lysosome or storage body is produced at the Golgi complex. Its genesis parallels that of secretory granules (Chaps. 3 and 21) in that its protein is synthesized in rough ER, is conveyed to the Golgi complex by transport vesicles, and in the Golgi complex it is cross-linked and aggregated, and

carbohydrate is added (see preceding section on Golgi Complex). Novikoff and his colleagues believe that lysosomes may also be produced in Golgi-associated ER, bypassing the Golgi complex proper, and they have coined the acronym "GERL complex" to encompass these cooperating structures. Primary lysosomes move to phagosomes and pinosomes and fuse with them to form secondary lysosomes, heterolysosomes, heterophagosomes, or heteropinosomes (Fig. 1–53), as described in the preceding section on smooth and coated vesicles. After fusion, the lysosomal enzymes mix with and digest the contents of the pinosomes or phagosomes. The low molecular-weight digestion products diffuse out of the lysosome into the surrounding cytoplasm where they are metabolized. Heterolysosomes may be long-lived and new endocytized material added over time. Heterolysosomes, moreover, may fuse with one another and form rather large, irregular complexes. Lysosomes finally reach a state in which the material they contain is not further degradable and their enzymatic capacity declines. They become residual bodies or telolysosomes. They may contain pigments, myelin bodies, crystals, lipids, and assorted materials. Residual bodies may be expelled from macrophages and from invertebrate cells, as amebocytes (exocytosis). Alternatively, they may accumulate in the cytoplasm as indices of "wear and tear" of aging, as exemplified by lipofuscin granules. Residual bodies, as expected, are notable in long-lived metabolically active cells, such as nerve cells and muscle cells.

Another group of secondary lysosomes consists of autophagocytic vacuoles or cytolysosomes. These vacuoles are heterolysosomes that contain some organelles of the cell such as mitochondria and ribosomes. They may originate from segments of smooth ER that curve around some cytoplasm and fuse to enclose it in a vacuole. These vacuoles may then fuse with primary lysosomes just as phagosomes do. Another mechanism accounting for their origin may be the incorporation of some cytoplasm directly into a lysosome. The formation of autophagosomes is a mechanism of "internal policing" of a cell that removes damaged or senescent cell substance. Autophagocytic vacuoles increase in starvation and aging and after tissue injury. They participate in the normal turnover of cell organelles by destroying the aged ones. Thus, mitochondria have a half-life of only 10 days in rat hepatocytes. They are removed by autophagy. Autophagocytic vacuoles form residual bodies.

Lysosomes have other metabolic functions. They may function in the degradation of glycogen. Evidence for this role comes from a type of glycogen storage disease, an illness of children characterized by a marked increase in liver size (hepatomegaly) due to the accumulation of glycogen. In this disease, lysosomes are deficient in *glycosidase*, the enzyme responsible for glycogen breakdown. Lysosomes function to regulate hormone production by *crinophagy*. The thyroid hormone *thyroxin* is produced as a conjugate of globulin. Its separation or hydrolysis from globulin seems to depend on incorporation of the thyroglobulin into lysosomes and hydrolysis by their hydrolytic enzymes. The destruction of excess mammotrophic hormone in the secretory cells of the pituitary gland and of parathyroid hormone in the secretory cells of the parathyroid gland is accomplished by autophagy of secretory granules (crinography).

Unlike secretory granules, lysosomes are typically not released but remain within the cytoplasm. Their genesis is parallel to that of secretory granules, however. In their synthesis in rough ER and Golgi complex, lysosomal enzymes retain phosphorylated mannose residues which interact with membrane receptors in the Golgi complex to induce the formation of membrane-bounded lysosomes which remain within the cytoplasm indefinitely (See discussion in Chapter 21). In the case of secretory proteins, on the other hand, the phosphorylated mannose residues are cleaved off in the ER or Golgi, leading to the formation of membrane-bounded secretory granules which do not remain within the cytoplasm but move to the cell surface and are secreted. In some instances, however, lysosomes may be secreted. Thus, transformed platelets plugging a tear in a blood vessel secrete lysosomes (lambda granules) and lysosome-related vesicles (alpha granules), which intensify blood coagulation. Osteoclasts lying on bone that is undergoing lysis seal off an area by sheetlike cytoplasmic processes whose edges attach to the bone. They then secrete their bone-dissolving lysosomal enzymes into this sealed pouch and thereby remove bone with great precision. A number of lysosome-associated diseases have been identified. The lysosomal membrane in leukocytes in Chediak-Higashi disease is abnormally resistant to fusion with phagosomes. Phagocytized bacteria are therefore not exposed to the lysosome's lytic enzymes; the cell's capacity to destroy bacteria is impaired, and affected individuals die of infection. More than 20 *storage diseases* due to deficient activity of lysosomal enzymes have been identified. In *Hurler's syndrome* connective tissue matrix accumulates because lysosomes fail to degrade acid mucopolysaccharides. The enlarged spleen (splenomegaly) and other pathology of *Gaucher's disease* seem to be due to a defect in lysosomal β-glucosidase. In glycogen-storage disease type II, α-glycosidase is absent from lysosomes so that hepatocytes (and the whole liver) become enlarged by stored glycogen-filled vesicles that cannot be metabolized. A contrasting group of lysosomal diseases is due to intracellular breakup of lysosomes. In gout, as a result of genetically induced high levels of uric acid in the body fluids, urate crystals form in the synovial cavities and other connective tissue spaces. Leukocytes engulf these crystals. As the crystals become incorporated into secondary lysosomes they disrupt the lysosomes, loosing the hydrolytic enzymes. The leukocytes are destroyed and the enzymes, released to the tissue, induce inflammation characteristic of gouty arthritis. This sequence may occur in asbestos intoxication, in experimentally induced methylcellulose disease, and in other instances in which lysosomes are confronted with irritating materials that they are unable to degrade.

Peroxisomes, or *microbodies of Rouiller* are involved in H_2O_2 metabolism. They are membrane-bounded organelles, somewhat larger than primary lysosomes (Fig. 1–48) and may be continuous with tubules of smooth ER. Peroxisomes are relatively numerous in hepatocytes (Chap. 20), in renal tubular cells (Chap. 24), and in macrophages. They contain flavin enzymes, such as *urate oxidase* and D-*amino acid oxidase*, which produce H_2O_2 by using molecular oxygen as an oxidizing agent. Peroxisomes have a variegated granular internum and, in the hepatocyte and some other cell types, contain a crystalline component that represents urate oxidase. However, H_2O_2, although necessary in a number of cellular reactions and capable of killing microorganisms, is tolerated in only low concentration by cells. In a sequential action to their generation of H_2O_2, peroxisomes, because they contain the enzyme *catalase*, convert H_2O_2 to water. Peroxisomes are also associated with α-keto acid formation and thereby participate in forming glucose from lipids and other noncarbohydrate precursors, a process termed *gluconeogenesis*.

Multivesicular bodies (MVB) are membrane-bounded vesicles 0.5 to 1.0 μm in diameter that contain a number of small vesicles with a diameter of 50 to 75 nm. They may be found in most

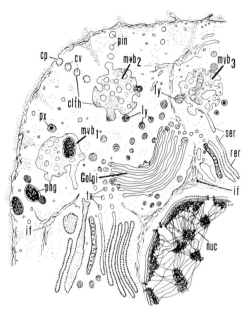

1–54 Multivesicular bodies **(mvb)** are prominent in this drawing. **mvb₁** contains a phagosome **(phg)**. **mvb₂** receives smooth **(pin)** and coated **(cv)** pinocytotic vesicles, the latter originating as coated pits **(cp)**. Plaques of clathrin **(clth)** lie on the surface of mvb₂ and mvb₃. Lysosomes fuse with mvb. **mvb₃**, containing mitochondria and rough ER **(rer)**, is autophagocytic. It is continuous with smooth ER **(ser)**. The Golgi complex is engaged in lysosome production and receives material from the ER in transport vesicles **(tv)**. Vimentin, a class of intermediate filament **(if)** surrounds the nucleus **(nuc)** and radiates in the cytoplasm.

cell types and are more numerous in cells rich in lysosomes. The membranes bounding MVB are usually smooth, but patches of their surface may be coated (see discussion of coated vesicles above). The MVB bounding membrane itself may invaginate and form some of the smaller vesicular structures and, like peroxisomes, may be continuous with short segments of smooth ER. Multivesicular bodies appear to represent reaction vats, receiving the contents of the endocytic vesicles and lysosomes that fuse with them. As a result, MVB possess the functions of a large heterolysosome. They may also receive the contents of secretory granules by crinophagy. They incorporate peroxisomes, partaking of their functions. Indeed, peroxisomes and other cellular structures may be autophagocytized in MVB (Fig. 1–54).

Microfilaments and Intermediate (100 Å) Filaments. There are two major groups of fine fila-

ments in virtually every cell type. One group is approximately 50 Å in diameter (Fig. 1–55) and is made of *actin*. These filaments, called *microfilaments,* are contractile and are believed to underlie the locomotion of cells, the ruffling and invagination of cell membranes, contraction, and other aspects of contractility. They form the terminal web of epithelial cells and enter microvilli. They also form the contractile ring in dividing cells (Fig. 1–55). They are best developed in muscle cells (Chap. 7). A second group of fine intracellular filaments is stouter, approximately 90 to 120 Å in diameter. They represent a more diverse population of filaments than the microfilaments and are referred to as *intermediate filaments or 100-Å filaments*. They possess mechanical functions in supporting or stiffening cells and in organizing intracellular organelles for coordinated activity.

Microfilaments are part of the actin–myosin system and become contractile by sliding over myosin filaments, as occurs in muscle cells. In nonmuscle cells actin, in the form of microfilaments, is visible by electron microscopy whereas myosin is not. Yet myosin is also present, as shown in a number of cell types by immunocytochemistry (Chap. 2). Thus, in the mitotic contractile ring in which actin microfilaments have been demonstrated by electron microscopy, the presence of myosin has been shown by fluorescence immunocytochemistry. It is likely that myosin is not visible in electron micrographs because it occurs in short segments representing oligomers, which aggregate into filaments only transiently or form filaments that our preparative methods fail to preserve. Furthermore, myosin is present in much lower concentration in most cells than actin. Its high concentration and layout in cells suggest that actin, in addition to its major contractile functions, has a cytoskeletal role. Actin can be detected by an excellent cytochemical test: its specific reaction with the S-1 subfraction of heavy meromyosin (HMM) (Fig. 1–55). The tissue is first extracted with glycerol to increase permeability and permit the penetrance of HMM. After irrigation with HMM, microfilaments become "decorated" with HMM, which gives them a characteristic fuzzy appearance resembling arrowheads. Actin may also be detected by more conventional immunocytochemical methods. Microfilaments are often concentrated at the surface of nonmuscle cells and, by high-resolution electron microscopy, appear to be attached to the cytoplasmic surface of the plasma membrane. Whether the microfilaments

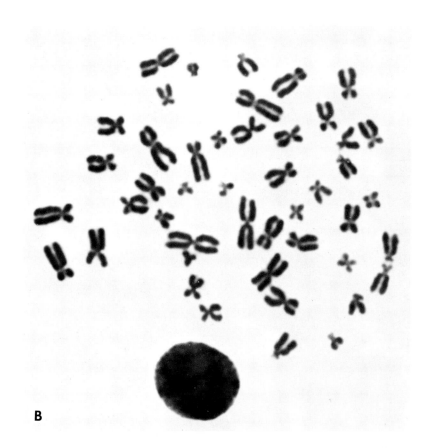

B

1–63 A. Human karyotype. Metaphase chromosomes have been arranged into morphologically similar groups of paired chromosomes and numbered. Pairs 1, 2, 3, and 16 can be identified as different from other chromosomes. It is impossible to separate 4 from 5, but 4 and 5 may be separated from the remainder. Similarly it is impossible to separate 6, 7, 8, 9, 10, 11, 12, and the X chromosome as different from one another, but this large group may be recognized as different from the other chromosomes. Chromosomes 13, 14, and 15, 17 and 18; 19 and 20 form similar groups. This individual is male, having an X and Y chromosome. **B.** The metaphase from which the karyotype was prepared. An interphase nucleus is present for comparison of size. Aceto-orcein stain. × 2,400. (From the work of B. Reuben Migeon.)

dense line transecting the cell. Viewed from one of the poles, the chromosomes form a circlet. Metaphase chromosomes are linear, densely stained structures. Each chromosome is constricted at one place along its length, an unstained zone called the *centromere* or *kinetochore*. The two chromatids of the chromosomes are free of one another except at the centromere, and the spindle fibers also attach there. Chromosomes may be divided into three groups, depending on the location of the centromere. If the centromere divides a chromosome into segments of equal length, the chromosome is *metacentric*. Those chromosomes separated into larger and smaller limbs by the centromere are *submedian*. Chromosomes in which the centromere is almost at the end, so that there is virtually only one limb, are *telocentric*.

The chromatic material of the chromosome may have another *secondary constriction* in one of the limbs. This constriction may have some length, and so it isolates the chromatic material

at the end of the chromosome into a *satellite*. Typically, nucleoli develop in certain zones of constriction in satellited chromosomes on reconstitution of daughter nuclei.

Metaphase chromosomes of each species may be classified on the basis of the location of the centromere, the size and shape of the limbs, and the presence of secondary constrictions and satellites. These characteristics make up the *karyotype,* or the morphology of the metaphase chromosomes. The karyotype of the human male is presented in Fig. 1–63A. The metaphase plate from which the karyotype was prepared is shown in Fig. 1–63B. The karyotype is prepared by cutting out the chromosome pairs from a photograph of a squash preparation of a metaphase cell selectively stained with a dye such as aceto-orcein. The cut-out chromosomes are then arranged in clusters of similar chromosomes. It is not possible to differentiate chromosomes occurring within a cluster by the standard aceto-orcein procedure. Thus, in the human male karyotype

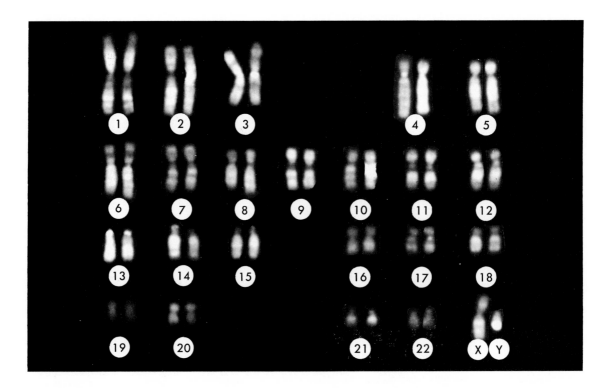

1–64 Karyotype of normal male (XY) cultured human leukocyte, showing quinacrine fluorescence patterns. Note the bandings present in each of the chromosomes. Although the significance of this banding is not understood, it has proved useful in differentiating chromosomes that are morphologically alike. Compare with the conventional karyotype in Fig. 1–63A and B. × 2,500. (From the work of W. R. Breg.) It has proved possible to obtain a similar banding pattern by staining a chromosomal preparation with a giemsa stain at a pH of about 6.8. The latter is a relatively easy procedure and may become more widely used than fluorescence staining.

one cannot separate chromosomes 6, 7, 8, 9, 10, 11, 12, and the X chromosome from one another. Certain fluorochromes produce a banded staining pattern in each of the chromosomes (Fig. 1–64). The banding pattern can also be shown in a more stable preparation by staining a squash preparation of a metaphase cell with dilute giemsa stain at pH 6.8. By this means it has proved possible to identify chromosomes not differentiable otherwise. Correlations of genetic diseases such as Down's syndrome (mongolism) and leukemia with abnormal karyotypes are being made in increasing number.

At the beginning of metaphase, the chroma-tids of a chromosome are connected only at the centromere. At the end of metaphase the centromeres divide and each of the chromatids, now a daughter chromosome and attached to the spindle by its own centromere, moves outward from the metaphase plate toward one pole of the cell. Thus, in human somatic cells, one set of 46 chromosomes moves to one centriole and the other set to the other. This divergent movement constitutes the *anaphase* of mitosis (Figs. 1–61, 1–62, and 1–65C). The spindle fibers attached to the centromeres are responsible for the characteristic orderly diverging movement of the chromosomes in anaphase. The drug colchicine interferes with the spindle by breaking up microtubules, leaving dividing cells suspended in metaphase and unable to complete the cell division.

Anaphase is concluded when the two chromosomal masses have moved to opposite poles of the cell. There now begins the final stage of nuclear division, *telophase* (Figs. 1–61, 1–62, and 1–65), during which two daughter nuclei are formed. Nuclear membranes form around each of the chromosomal masses, nucleoli appear at the satellite-bearing chromosomes, and segments of the chromosomes uncoil to become euchromatin.

Although primary attention must be accorded

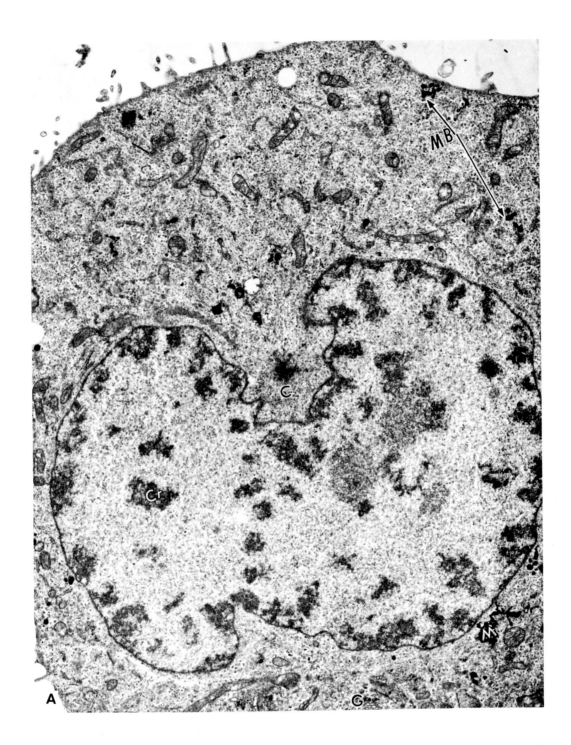

1–65 **A–D** Electron micrograph of mitosis in a human HeLa cell in tissue culture. These cells, originally derived from a carcinoma of the uterine cervix, form a strain of cells maintained in tissue culture. **A.** In early prophase, the chromatin becomes clumped because of the condensation of chromosomes **(Cr).** The nuclear membrane is still intact, and the centriole **(C)** and multivesicular bodies **(MB)** are prominent. Approximately × 3,850. (From Robbins, E., and Gonatas, N. K. 1964. J. Cell Biol. 21:429.)

(continued)

72

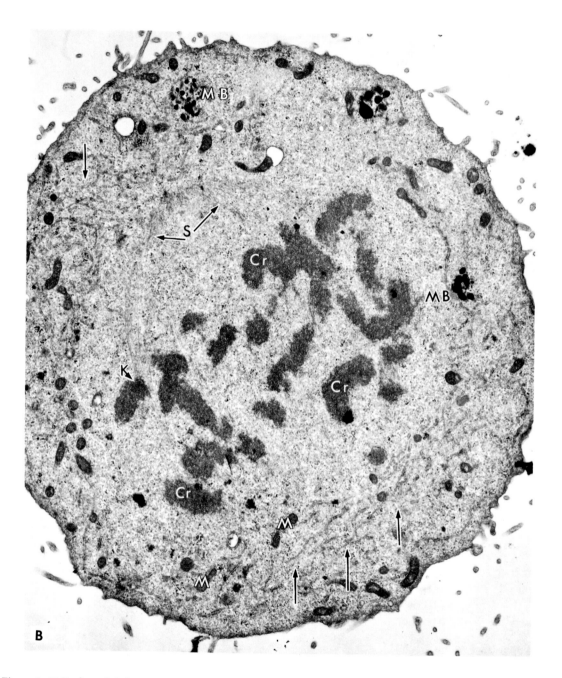

Figure 1–65 B △ and C ▷

C. In late anaphase, the two chromosomal masses
have moved apart. They are already surrounded by a
double nuclear membrane. At the lower pole, a
portion of a centriole and spindle fibers may be seen.
Note how the spindle fibers are present, together with
some mitochondria, in the constriction between what
will be the two daughter cells. Note, too, the blebs of
cytoplasm **(BL)** about the periphery of the se cells,
indicating the frothing that occurs in this phase.
Approximately × 5,225. (From Robbins, E., and
Gonatas, N. K. 1964. J. Cell Biol. 21:429.)

B. In later prophase the chromosomes are close to the
equatorial plate and metaphase. The spindle fibers **(S)**
are seen radiating from the centriole and attached to a
chromosome at the kinetochore **(K).** Approximately
× 5,640. (From Robbins, E., and Gonatas, N. K. 1964.
J. Cell Biol. 21:429.)

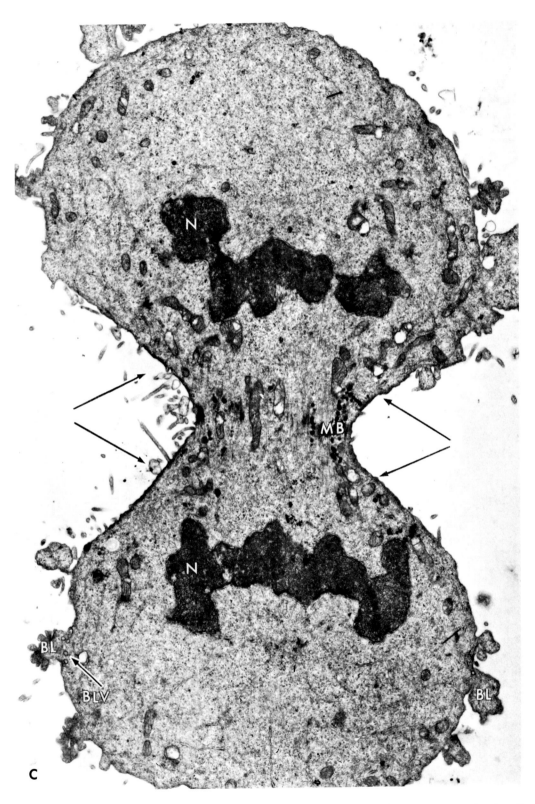

(continued)

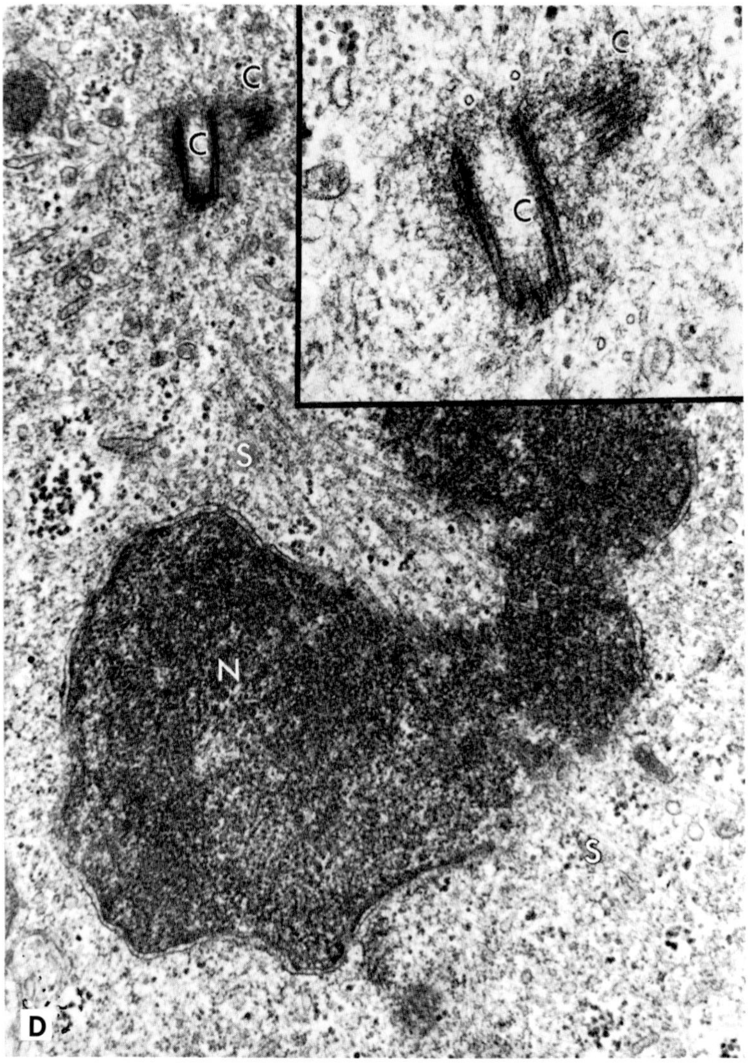

Figure 1–65D
D. Telophase. Note the presence of a double nuclear membrane about a daughter nucleus. The centriole (at higher magnification in the inset) has already been duplicated. Approximately × 13,750 (inset × 30,800). (From Robbins, E., and Gonatas, N. K. 1964. J. Cell Biol. 21:429.)

the nucleus in mitosis, characteristic changes occur in the cytoplasm. The division of the centrioles and the formation of the achromatic apparatus in prophase have already been discussed. Frothing or bubbling of the cytoplasm occurs in anaphase. During this bubbling phase, the cell surfaces are covered with microvilli. Indeed, microvilli occur throughout mitosis, being most prominent in anaphase. They also occur during G, but are usually absent or scanty in the rest of the cell cycle (Fig. 1–70). With the separation of the nuclear masses in anaphase, a partition of cytoplasmic constituents occurs. Mitochondria, lysosomes, ribosomes, and cytoplasmic membranes become distributed in

approximately equal amounts about the two newly formed nuclei. As the nuclear membrane is reconstructed, the cytoplasm becomes deeply constricted in a *constriction ring* (Figs. 1–55 and 1–65C) between the two masses of chromosomes. The cytoplasm divides, forming two equal daughter cells. For a short time, the spindle may persist as a transient bridge between daughter cells.

Amitosis. Amitosis may occur in terminal or highly transient cell types such as certain cells of the placenta or of the blood. It may also occur in some multinucleated cells, as the giant cells of the connective tissue. In amitosis the nuclear

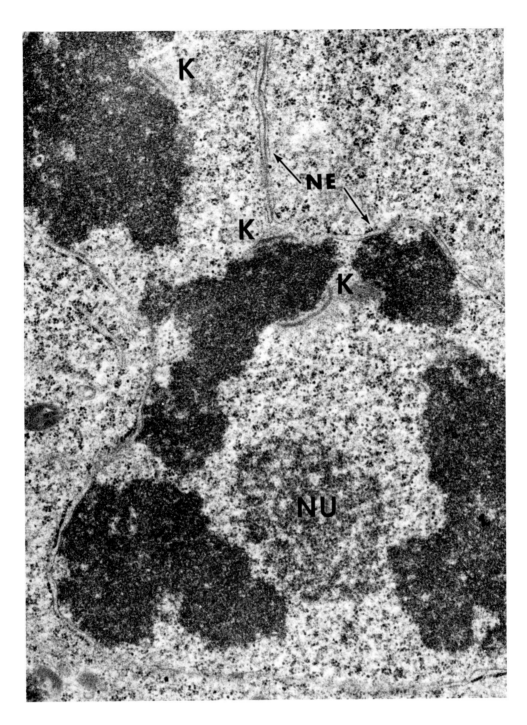

membrane appears to constrict deeply and a single nucleus becomes pinched into two. Although equal-sized daughter nuclei may sometimes result, it is impossible that a precise separation of chromosomal material can be achieved (Fig. 1–71).

1–66 Later prophase. Chinese hamster fibroblast. Fully formed kinetochores **(K)** and a nucleus **(NU)** are present. The nuclear envelope **(NE)** is almost completely intact. [From Brinkley, B. R., and Stubblefield, E. 1970. *In* D. M. Prescott, L. Goldstein, and E. McConkey (eds.)]

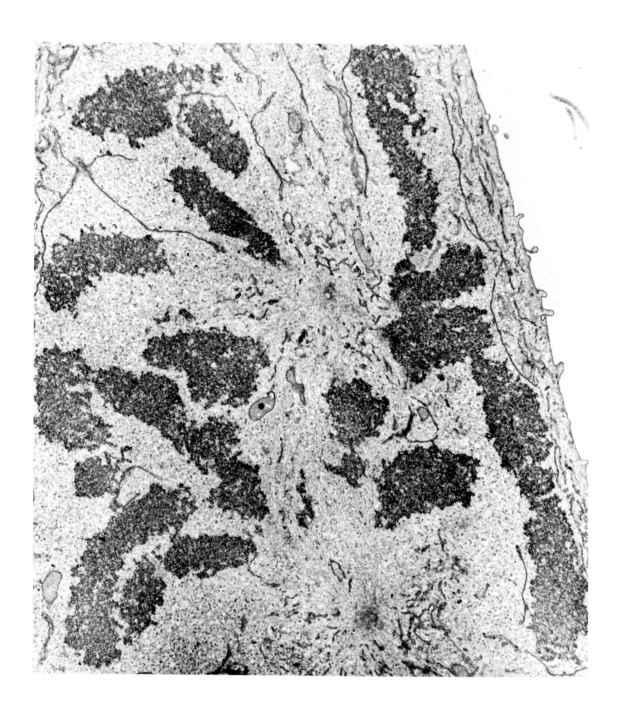

1–67 Prometaphase, rat kangaroo fibroblast. Here each of the chromosomes is tightly coiled and, although not evident, split into two chromatids. The chromosomes are moving to take positions on the metaphase plate. A centriole and microtubules are present in the cytoplasm. × 14,000. (From the work of B. R. Brinkley.)

Polyteny and Poliploidy. DNA replication may occur without nuclear division. It is characteristic of certain cell types, such as the salivary gland cells of diptera, that DNA replication occurs without subsequent chromosomal division, resulting in *polytene* chromosomes. These chromosomes replicate themselves many times over. However, the replicates remain together

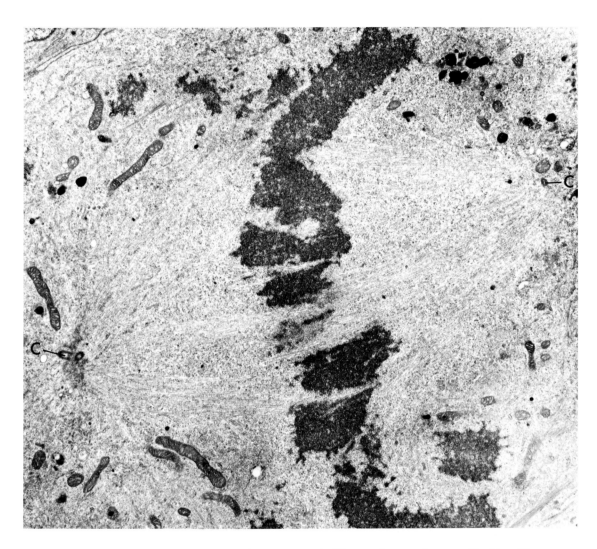

rather than move apart into separate chromosomes and thereby form giant chromosomes. Polytenic chromosomes readily show a type of banding that requires fluorochromes or special giemsa staining (Fig. 1–64) to demonstrate in other chromosomes.

DNA replication may occur with subsequent chromosomal duplication but without loss of nuclear membranes or karyokinesis, resulting in polyploid nuclei. The process has been termed *endomitosis*. Polyploid nuclei thus contain multiples of the diploid number of chromosomes. They are typically larger than diploid nuclei, as in some hepatocytes and megakaryocytes.

Meiosis. Meiosis is a type of nuclear division, restricted to gametes (i.e., spermatocytes and

1–68 Metaphase, rat kangaroo fibroblast. The metaphase plate is present in edge-on view. On the left, two centrioles **(C)** may be observed; on the right, one centriole. The microtubules of the spindle radiate from the centrioles. Both chromosomal (attached to kinetochore) and continuous (pole to pole) microtubules are present. × 10,350. (From Brinkley, B. R., and Cartwright, J., Jr. 1971. J. Cell Biol. 50:416.)

oocytes) wherein the number of chromosomes characteristic of somatic cells, the *diploid* number (2n), is halved to the *haploid* number (1n). This halving occurs because the homologs in each chromosome pair separate from one another. Each daughter nucleus in meiosis contains a set of homologs. For this reason, meiosis is called *reduction division*. The haploid nuclei of

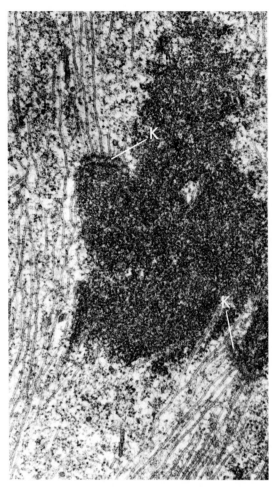

1–69 Metaphase, rat kangaroo fibroblast.
Chromosomal microtubules are inserted into kinetochores **(K).** Note the double nature of the kinetochore. Continuous microtubules pass between the chromosomes running from pole to pole without insertion into kinetochores. × 30,800. (From Brinkley, B. R., and Cartwright, J., Jr. 1971. J. Cell Biol. 50:416.)

the gametes unite and the diploid number of chromosomes is restored in the process of fertilization. The fertilized ovum and all its somatic descendants divide by mitotic division, and the diploid number is thereby maintained in somatic cells. But meiosis has the second major function of providing genetic variation by the exchange of segments between homologous chromosomes and the random selection of one of the two homologs during the reduction division into a given daughter nucleus.

Meiosis involves two successive nuclear divisions with only one division of chromosomes (Figs. 1–72 and 1–73). The first meiotic division is characterized by a prolonged prophase. In this prophase the homologous chromosomes come to lie together, closely and exactly paired in a point-for-point correspondence along their entire length *(synapsis).* During the process the chromosomes shorten by coiling, but not as much as in the prophase of mitosis. Moreover, each of the chromosomes is observed to be longitudinally split into two chromatids. The homologous paired chromosomes, termed a *bivalent,* therefore consist of four chromatids. A spindle forms and the bivalents arrange themselves on a metaphase plate. The divergent movement of anaphase begins as the homologs, consisting of two chromatids each, move apart to opposite poles and are then separated into daughter cells at telophase. Thenceforth, after the first meiotic division, each of the daughter cells contains one of the homologous chromosomes split into two chromatids. It is of great significance that in the first meiotic division the kinetochore does not divide, as it does in mitosis, and so the chromatids remain together. A second meiotic division ensues in which the chromosomes become arranged in a metaphase plate and the kinetochores divide. The chromatids that make up each of the chromosomes are now free of one another and diverge from the metaphase plate in an anaphase movement. Later in telophase they are grouped into daughter nuclei and then daughter cells. The two meiotic divisions have thus sorted the four homologous chromatids present in prophase of the first meiotic division into four separate gametes, each of which has the haploid number of chromosomes. In a male, four functional spermatozoa will result from the two meiotic divisions. Curiously, the completion of cytokinesis in the spermatozoa is delayed so that four otherwise mature spermatozoa may remain linked in Siamese-quadruplet style. In a female four ova are produced as well, but the cytoplasmic division leaves virtually all the cytoplasm with one nucleus. The remaining nuclei, surrounded by minimal cytoplasm, cannot survive. They are called *polar bodies.* This unequal cytoplasmic division provides one nucleus with sufficient cytoplasm to support fertilization and embryogenesis. Each of the gamete nuclei contains 23 chromosomes. In female gametes one of these is an X chromosome, whereas in male ga-

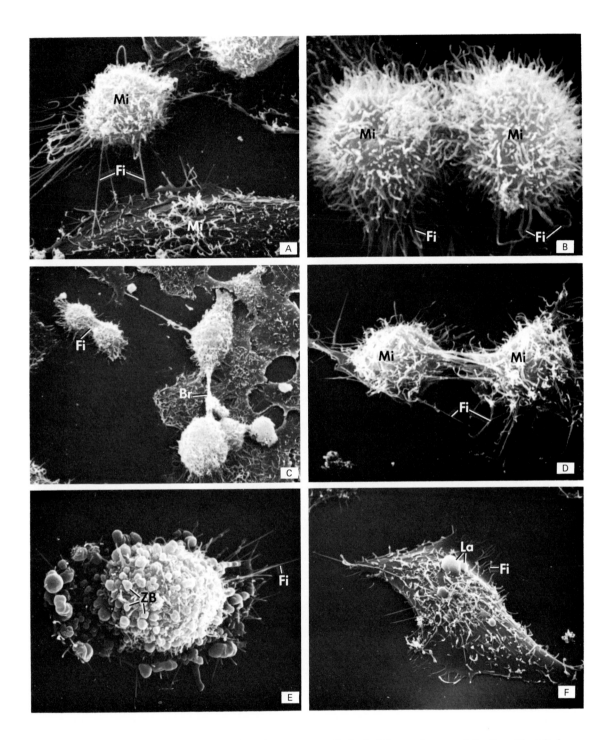

1–70 Scanning electron microscopy of cultured HeLa **(A, C, and F)** and KB cells **(B, D, and E)** in mitosis. Late stages in cell division are illustrated in B to D; interphase cells are illustrated in C, E, and F. Note the long bridge **(Br)** connecting the daughter cells in C. Other surface specializations identified are microvilli **(Mi)**, filopodia **(Fi)**, lamellapodia **(La)**, and blebs **(ZB)**. A, × 1,664; B, × 3,600; C, × 684; D, × 2,040; E, × 1,889; F, × 1,680. (From Beams, H. W., and Kessel, R. G. 1976. Am. Sci. 64:279.)

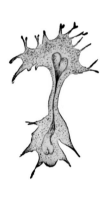
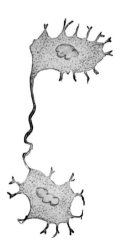
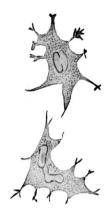

1–71 Amitosis in a histiocyte of a frog. The drawing is prepared from a cell in tissue culture. (From the work of Arnold.)

metes one is either an X or a Y. During fetal life in a human female, oocytes migrate into the ovary, proliferate by mitosis a short time, and then undergo meiosis, entering the prophase of the first meiotic division. They remain in that state until shortly before ovulation. Because a woman may ovulate until about 45 years of age, oocytes may remain in meiosis for more than 45 years. It may well be that the first meiotic prophase constitutes a particularly stable state for DNA.

Another essential function of meiosis is to provide genetic variation. It will be recalled that in diploid cells one chromosome in a homologous pair is contributed by the spermatozoon and the other by the oocyte. When the homologous chromosomes are arranged on the first meiotic metaphase plate, it is a matter of chance whether the homolog contributed by the sperm or the homolog contributed by the ovum faces a given pole. As a result, in each cell produced in the first meiotic division, the proportion of chromosomes derived from the sperm and that from

the egg are a matter of chance. This chance separation is one mechanism of genetic mixture. A second mechanism is the exchange, by homologous chromosomes, of corresponding segments. This exchange occurs when the homologs are in synapsis during the early phases of meiotic prophase I (Fig. 1–73). The extent of the exchange becomes apparent as the homologs pull away from their synaptic union. It is then seen that they frequently remain attached in one or more places. This persistent link between diverging chromosomes is termed a *chiasma*. The exchange of segments is termed *crossing over*.

The stages in meiosis are as follows (Fig. 1–72):

1. The first prophase, prophase I, is long and may be divided into five stages. In *leptotene* the chromosomes are long and thin. In *zygotene* the homologous chromosomes move toward one another and pair, lying in close touch in a point-for-point correspondence along their length (synapsis). In *pachytene* the

1–72 The stages of meiosis I and II shown schematically. A pair of homologous chromosomes, one dark and the other light, is followed through meiosis I. Then chromatids of a daughter cell are traced through meiosis II. The events are as follows:

Prophase I. Leptotene: The chromosomes become apparent as thin linear structures. Zygotene: Homologous chromosomes line up and pair with one another point to point (synapsis). Pachytene: With pairing completed, the chromosomes become shorter and thicker and each longitudinally splits into chromatids, the centromere remaining single. The four

chromatids of the two chromosomes constitute a bivalent. Chromatids from each of the homologous chromosomes may cross over one another forming a chiasma. Diplotene: The chromosomes further shorten and broaden; they also coil. Homologous chromosomes begin to move apart but are held together at the chiasma. Diakinesis: The chromosomes become broader, thicker, more tightly coiled; they move further apart.

- Metaphase I. The chromosomes are on the equatorial plate.
- Anaphase I. The chromosomes diverge, exchanging chromosomal segments at the site of the chiasma.

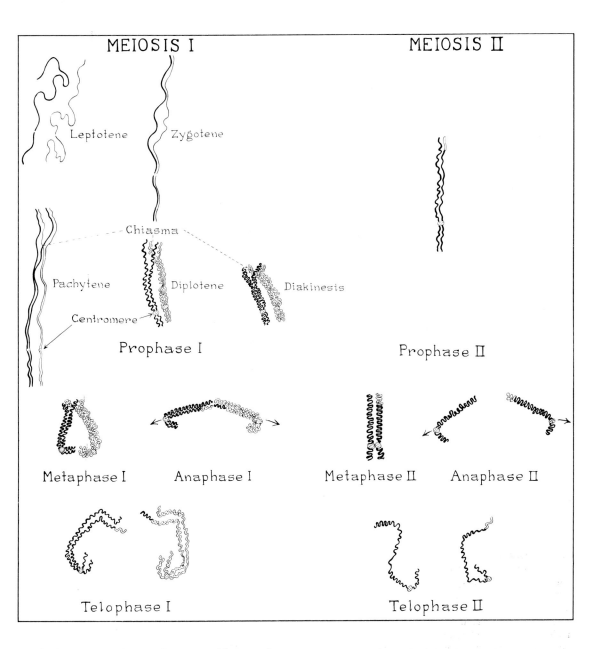

MEIOSIS I   MEIOSIS II

Leptotene   Zygotene

Chiasma

Pachytene   Diplotene   Diakinesis

Centromere

Prophase I   Prophase II

Metaphase I   Anaphase I   Metaphase II   Anaphase II

Telophase I   Telophase II

- Telophase I. Each chromatid pair joined by a single centromere, lies in a daughter cell. The chromatids uncoil and lengthen to some extent.
- Chromatids in the left-hand daughter cell pass through the following stages in meiosis II.
- Prophase II. This stage is transient and possibly absent since the chromatids may move directly to metaphase II.
- Metaphase II. Chromatids become shorter, broader, and coiled. The centromere divides.
- Anaphase II. Chromatids separate and move to opposite poles.

- Telophase II. Each of the chromatids is now a daughter cell.

Thus in the course of these two divisions the four chromatids forming the bivalent of prophase I are separated, first into two daughter cells of telophase I, each containing two chromatids (4n → 2n), and then into two daughter cells again in telophase II, each containing one chromatid (2n → 1n). A total of four daughter cells is produced each having the haploid (1n) number of chromosomes. In a male individual four sperms are produced; in a female, one ovum and three polar bodies. On fertilization the diploid (2n) number is restored.

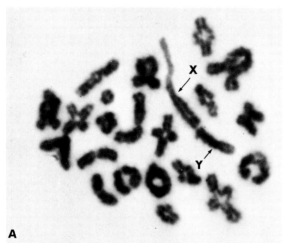

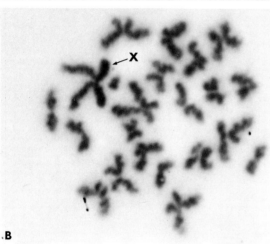

1-73 Meiosis in the golden hamster *Mesocricetus auratus*. **A.** Primary spermatocyte showing the 22 bivalents at the first meiotic metaphase. The X and Y chromosomes are associated terminally, the X being distinguished by its length. The autosomal bivalents demonstrate chiasmata in various stages. Note the coiling of the chromatids. **B.** Secondary spermatocyte at the second meiotic metaphase, containing the haploid number of 22 chromosomes. This cell has received the Y chromosome. At this stage, the chromosomes show "relic" spirals, which are probably remnants of coiling from the first meiotic division. Aceto-orcein stain. × 2,200. (From the work of M. Fergusen-Smith.)

chromosomes coil considerably, appearing shorter and thicker. At about this time it becomes apparent that each of the chromosomes of the bivalent contains four chromatids. The centromere does not split. In *diplotene* the chromosomes begin to separate from one an-

other, but the separation is incomplete, with chiasmata forming. The separation continues into the *diakinesis*, a stage that shows the chiasmata and the thickened, coiled, partially separated chromosomes to good advantage. The nuclear membrane disappears.

2. In metaphase I the bivalent chromosomes are arranged on an equatorial plate. There are two centromeres, one for each of the chromosomes, and the centromeres are attached to spindle fibers.
3. In anaphase I the chromosomes, each of which consists of two chromatids, move to opposite poles.
4. Telophase I follows, but the chromosomes may remain in a shortened form.

In the first meiotic division, therefore, the diploid number of chromosomes has been reduced to the haploid number; an exchange of genetic information may have occurred between the chromosomes; the distribution of chromosomes of a given bivalent to each pole has been a matter of chance, further increasing genetic variation; and each of the chromosomes is longitudinally split to form two chromatids.

5. Interphase, or *interkinesis*, is brief.
6. In prophase II a spindle forms, the nuclear membrane breaks down, and the chromosomes move equatorially.
7. In metaphase II the chromatids are arranged on an equatorial plate and their centromeres divide and become attached to spindle fibers.
8. In anaphase II the chromatids, now daughter chromosomes, move to opposite poles.
9. Telophase II is marked by the appearance of a nuclear membrane uncoiling of the chromosomes, and the development of daughter cells.

The Life Cycle of Cells

Two major types of cell may be recognized: *somatic cells*, which are the diverse cells making up the somatic structure of the body, fated to die with or before the individual they constitute; and *germ cells*, which are the gametes capable of uniting sexually with those of another individual to form a new individual.

A somatic cell begins its life span as one of the daughter cells of a mitotic division. Directly after this division the cell may undergo a period of intense protein synthesis, resulting in the emergence of the granules, filaments, or other specific structures that mark the cell as mature and specialized. As the cell matures and morphological signs of specialization occur, it is differentiated from an unspecialized, perhaps multipotential, cell into a highly specialized unit of limited cellular potency. Although a cell may appear undifferentiated, its direction of maturation may be fixed and limited genetically, only time being required to disclose the nature of the differentiation by the appearance of morphological specializations. In short, a cell that appears morphologically undifferentiated may, in fact, be quite specifically determined.

The frequency of mitotic division varies with the cell type and tissue. Tissues may be classified as showing no mitotic division, resulting in no renewal (nervous tissue); little division, resulting in slow renewal (liver and thyroid); and active division, resulting in fast renewal (gastrointestinal tract and hematopoietic tissue). Some slowly renewed tissues may be termed "conditional renewal" systems because their renewal rate can be considerably increased under certain circumstances. After partial hepatectomy, for example, the remaining hepatocytes divide very actively, providing fast renewal until the mass of the liver is restored. Even some cells showing no mitotic division may, with appropriate stimulation, proliferate and differentiate. Certain small lymphocytes (T cells) may circulate and recirculate for many years in humans without dividing, but when stimulated by the appropriate antigen, or with certain mitogens, such as phytohemagglutinin or pokeweed, they may divide rapidly, producing clones of immunologically competent cells. In neurons, mitosis occurs only prenatally and neonatally until the full number of neurons is reached. Thereafter, no replacement occurs; a cell lost diminishes the total number, and its absence may cause functional impairment. The cells in tissues undergoing slow renewal tend to be long-lived. The relatively low levels of mitotic division provide new cells to replace those dying off or to permit the growth and increased functional capacity of the tissue. Rapidly renewing tissues are characterized by short-lived cells replaced by cell division, so that a rather stable number of cells results. In the intestinal epithelium, new cells formed in the depths of the intestinal glands appear to move up the wall of the gland replacing the topmost cells, which fall into the gut lumen. As a result, the entire intestinal epithelium is renewed in a span of days. The kinetics of hematopoietic tissues, particularly of the granular leukocytes, follows this pattern.

It is possible to define a *generation time* for a population of similar cells, relating the interphase state, the period of DNA replication, and the process of mitotic division. A series of three periods follows mitosis: G_1, S, G_2, then M. G_1 is an interval or gap that follows cell division; S is the period of DNA replication; G_2 is the gap between replication of DNA and the start of mitosis; and M is mitosis.

The duration of G_1 varies greatly with cell types and mitotic turnover. In rapidly dividing cells it may be a matter of several hours. In nonrenewing tissues it may last the life of the organism. Such prolonged G_1 periods may be designated G_0. S is demonstrated by autoradiography. Thymidine is a base distinctive to DNA. Therefore, replicating DNA specifically and selectively takes up thymidine. If the thymidine is radioactive, accomplished by the incorporation of tritium (^{3}H) in the molecule, and is administered during DNA replication, it is taken up by the replicating DNA and can mark it in autoradiographs. Indeed, the ability to delineate the S period by this means makes it possible to determine the entire generation time. In a rapidly renewing tissue, S is approximately 7 h. It is a matter of great interest that the DNA in a given chromosome does not all replicate at the same time. Instead, different segments of the chromosome replicate at different times in the S period, and in a characteristic sequence. G_2 is very short—about an hour—in rapidly renewing tissues. In cells destined to be polytenic, G_2 may last indefinitely. The whole of the cycle in such rapidly dividing rodent tissues as germinal centers or thymus may be about 12 h. In the epithelium of the gastrointestinal tract in humans G_2 is 1 to 7 h.; the S phase, 10 to 20 h; G_1, 10 to 20 h; and the whole of the cycle, 1 to 2 days. In rodents this cycle may take only a third of this time.

The sequences in the generation cycle may be illustrated as follows[2]:

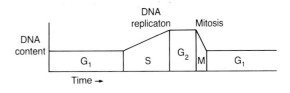

---

[2]After Lamerton, L. F., 1969, *In* Fry, R. J. M., Griem, M. L., and Kirsten, W. H. (eds.), Normal and Malignant Cell Growth. New York: Springer-Verlag.

After functioning as a mature cell for varying lengths of time, a cell dies, its death often presaged by a period of senescence. Perhaps the best-studied case is that of the erythrocyte, whose life span in the circulation of humans is approximately 120 days. Near the end of its life span, the activity of glucose-6-phosphatase and certain other enzymes declines, and the cell becomes mechanically more fragile. There are, however, no morphological concomitants of erythrocyte senescence.

In other cell types, however, morphological changes may signify senescence and coming cell death. In muscle cells, these changes include attenuation, decrease in specific functional elements such as contractile filaments, and accumulation of pigment. Other changes include diminution in mitochondria, accumulation of fat, and vacuolization of cytoplasm and nucleus. Dead cells may disappear by lysis, by phagocytosis, or by displacement from the tissue, seen in desquamated skin cells and intestinal cells.

References and Selected Bibliography

General

Baker, J. R. 1958. Principles of Biological Microtechnique: A Study of Fixation and Dyeing. New York: John Wiley and Sons, Inc.

Baker, J. R. The cell-theory: A restatement, history and critique. Q. J. Microbiol. Sci. 89:103 (1948); 90:87 (1949); 93:157 (1952).

Bensley, R. R., and Gersh I. 1933. Studies on cell structure by the freezing-drying method. I. Introduction. II. The nature of the mitochondria in the hepatic cell of amblystoma. III. The distribution in cells of the basophil substances, in particular the Nissl substance of the nerve cell. Anat. Rec. 57:205, 217, 369.

Bensley, R. R., and Hoerr, N. L. 1935. Studies on cell structure by the freezing-drying method. VI. The preparation and properties of mitochondria. Anat. Rec. 60:449.

Bodmer, W. F. 1981. The HLA system: Introduction. Brit. Med. Bull. 34:213.

Brachet, J., and Mirsky, A. E. (eds.). 1961. The cell. I. Biochemistry, physiology, morphology. II. Cells and their component parts. III. Mitosis and meiosis. IV. Specialized cells, pt. 1. V. Specialized cells, pt. 2. New York: Adademic Press, Inc.

Busch, H. B. (ed.). 1974. The Cell Nucleus. 3 vols. New York: Academic Press.

De Robertis, E. D. F., Saez, F. A., and De Robertis, E. M. F., Jr. 1975. Cell Biology, 6th ed. Philadelphia: W. B. Saunders Co.

Freeman, J. A., and Spurlock, B. O. 1962. A new epoxy embedment for electron microscopy. J. Cell Biol. 13:437.

Fuks, A., Kaufman, J. F., Orr, H. T., Parham, P., Robb, R. R., Terhorst, C., and Strominger, J. L. 1980. Structural aspects of the products of the human histocompatibility complex. Transplant. Proc. 9:1685.

Harris, H. 1974. Nucleus and Cytoplasm, 3rd ed. New York: Oxford University Press.

Karp, G. 1979. Cell Biology. New York: McGraw-Hill Book Co., Inc.

Organization of the Cytoplasm. 1982. Cold Spring Harbor Symp. Quant. Biol. Vol. 46.

Pretlow, T. G. II., Weir, E. E., and Zettergren, J. G. 1975. Problems connected with the separation of different kinds of cells. Int. Rev. Exp. Pathol. 14:91.

Siegel, B. M. (ed.). 1964. Modern developments in electron microscopy. In The Physics of the Electron Microscope: Techniques: Applications. New York: Academic Press, Inc.

Watson, D. D. 1976. Molecular Biology of the Gene, 3rd ed. New York: Benjamin.

Cell Cycle, Mitosis, and Centrioles

Ackerman, G. A. 1961. Histochemistry of the centrioles and centrosomes of the leukemic cells from human myeloblastic leukemia. J. Biophys. Biochem. Cytol. 11:717.

Bajer, A., and Mole-Bajer, 1971. Architecture and function of the mitotic spindle. Adv. Cell Mol. Biol. 1:213.

Baserga, R. (ed.). 1976. Multiplication and Division in Mammalian Cells. New York: Marcel Dekker.

Beams, W. H., and Kessel, R. G. 1976. Cytokinesis: A comparative study of cytoplasmic division in animal cells. Am. Sci. 64:279.

Brinkley, B. R., and Porter, K. R. (eds.). 1977. Symposium on "The Eukarocyte Cell Cycle." Inter. Cell Biol. New York: The Rockefeller Press, p. 409.

Brinkley, B. R., and Stubblefield, E. 1970. Ultrastructure and interaction of the kinetochore and centriole in mitosis and meiosis. In D. M. Prescott, L. Goldstein, and E. McConkey (eds.), Advances in Cell Biology, vol. I. New York: Appleton-Century-Crofts.

Bullough, W. S. 1975. Mitotic control in adult mammalian tissues. Biol. Rev. 50:99.

Edenberg, J., and Huberman, J. A. 1975. Eukaryotic chromosome replication. Ann. Rev. Genet. 9:245.

Fuge, H. 1974. Ultrastructure and function of the spindle apparatus and chromosomes during nuclear division. Protoplasm 82:299.

Gall, J. G., Porter, K. R., and Siekevitz, P. (eds.). 1981. Discovery in cell biology. J. Cell Biol. 91 (3, part 2):35.

Goss, R. T. 1970. Turnover in cells and tissues. In D. M. Prescott, L. Goldstein, and E. McConkey (eds.), Advances in Cell Biology, vol. 1. New York: Appleton-Century-Crofts, Inc.

Kornberg, A. DNA Synthesis. 1974. W. H. Freeman.

Lajtha, L. 1969. Proliferative capacity of hemopoietic stem cells. In R. J. M. Fry, M. G. Griem, and W. H. Kirsten (eds.), Normal and Malignant Cell Growth. New York: Springer-Verlag.

LeBlond, C. P., and Walker, B. E. 1956. Renewal of cell populations. Physiol. Rev. 36:255.

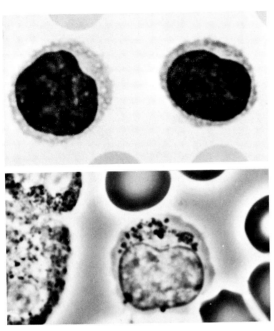

11–6 Lymphocytes of human blood. **Top.** Blood film
has been fixed and stained with Wright's
stain. Two small lymphocytes are present. **Bottom.**
Small blood lymphocyte is seen in a phase-contrast
photomicrograph. × 2,400. (From the work of G. A.
Ackerman.)

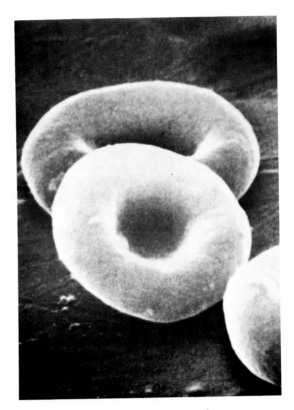

11–7 Human erythrocytes; scanning electron
micrograph × 10,000. (From Morel, F. M. M.,
Baker, R. F., and Wayland, H., 1971. J. Cell Biol.
48:91.)

Electron Microscopy of Blood Cells

In thin sections examined by transmission electron microscopy, erythrocytes contain a uniformly granular density representing hemoglobin. Some ferritin may be present. Ribosomes,
mitochondria, endoplasmic reticulum (ER), Golgi
complexes, and lysosomes are absent in mature
cells. Clear vesicles may be present. Spectrin, a
protein distinctive to erythrocytes, occurs as a
network of filaments beneath the plasma membrane. It may be masked in normal hemoglobin-
containing cells, but visible in hemolyzed cells.
The plasma membrane is trilaminar in section
(see Fig. 1–24) but contains many descrete structures shown in freeze-fracture etch preparations
(Fig. 1–26). In scanning electron microscopy
the biconcave shape of erythrocytes is striking
(Fig. 11–7).

Neutrophils (Fig. 11–8) possess two types of
granules that are membrane-bounded and together number about 200. *Primary, type A* granules, corresponding to the azurophilic granules
of light microscopy, account for about 20% of the
granules. They are relatively large (approximately 0.4 μm), dense, and homogeneous when
well fixed. Often some extraction occurs during
the processing, however, leaving less-dense irregular structures. Approximately 80% of the
granules are *definitive, secondary,* or *type B.*
They are smaller, less than 0.3 μm, less dense
than primary granules, and may contain a crystalloid (Fig. 11–8). Type B granules are often invisible by light microscopy so that only the relatively few azurophilic granules can be seen.[2]

---

[2]The term neutrophil designates the human cell. In rabbits
and certain other species, the secondary granules are eosinophilic, large, and spherical. In birds the granules are eosinophilic and rod-shaped. To distinguish these cells from true eosinophils, they are termed *pseudoeosinophils.* The generic
term for this cell type regardless of species and staining reaction is *heterophil.* By electron microscopy, heterophils of rabbits (pseudoeosinophils) and human beings (neutrophils) are
remarkably alike. But these terminological distinctions are
being lost in usage. The term heterophil is being used to refer
to those granulocytes, in birds, for example, that are the coun-
terparts of the neutrophil.

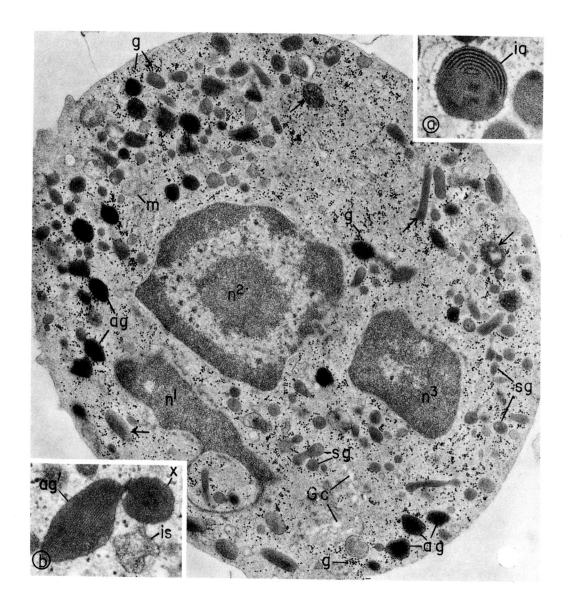

11–8 Mature human polymorphonuclear neutrophil (PMN). Several lobes of the nucleus are present (n^1 to n^3), and numerous granules, as well as glycogen (g), are scattered throughout the cytoplasm. A few mitochondria (m) and a small Golgi complex (Gc) are also visible. Some of the granules present are large and dense (ag), whereas others are small and less dense (sg). However, many granules are intermediate in size and density. Elongated forms, including football and dumbbell shapes, are also present (arrows). The insets depict internal structure within the large, dense (azurophilic) granules. **Inset a** shows a spherical granule (ia) containing concentric half-rings. **Inset b** illustrates the crystalline lattice with periodicity of approximately 100 Å, which is commonly seen in football or ellipsoid forms (ag'). A cross section (X) of the ellipsoid form and an immature specific granule (is) are also present in this field taken from a PMN myelocyte. The sequence of development of these cells together with additional electron micrographs (Fig. 12–15) is presented in Chaps. 12 and 13. **a,** × 45,000; **b,** × 45,000. (From Bainton, D. F., Ullyot, J. L., and Farquhar, M. G. 1971. J. Exp. Med. 134:907.)

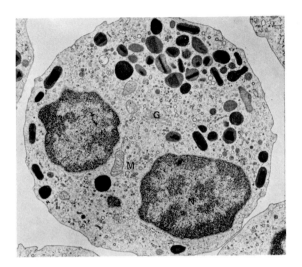

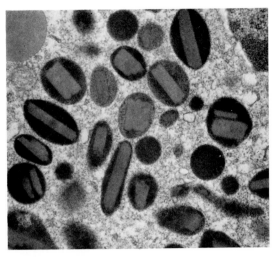

11–9 Eosinophil obtained from the peripheral blood of a normal human subject. Fixed with glutaraldehyde and osmium tetroxide. Note that the granules have an electron-dense "core" and a less electron-dense "matrix." **N**, bilobed nucleus; **G**, Golgi body; **M**, mitochondria. × 7,742. (From Zucker-Franklin, D. 1974. Adv. Intern. Med. 19:1.)

11–10 Eosinophil granules treated with phosphotungstic acid during dehydration. Note that the electron density of the core and matrix is reversed. × 27,160. (From Zucker-Franklin, D. 1974. Adv. Intern. Med. 19:1.)

Eosinophils have large (0.16 to 1.0 µm), spherical, membrane-bounded granules that contain an angular, dense, and lamellated crystalloid (Figs. 11–9 and 11–10). They also contain a few smaller dense nonspecific granules.

The specific granules of basophils are membrane-bounded structures about 0.5 µm in diameter (Fig. 11–11, A and B) that contain granular material, myelin figures, lucent zones, and crystalloids. A few nonspecific granules may also be present. Specific granules are similar but not identical to the granules of mast cells, (Chap. 4).

Lymphocytes (Figs. 11–12 and 11–13) contain a number of lysosomal granules and small-to-moderately sized Golgi complexes. They may contain polyribosomes and some profiles of smooth ER, but, unless undergoing "blast" transformation or proliferation (discussed under Lymphocytes, below), they possess little rough ER. Lymphocytes, as other cells, have distinctive molecules on their cell surface. They are not evident in conventional transmission electron micrographs, but may be visualized by special stains (see following section on Cytochemistry).

Monocytes contain moderate numbers of lysosomes, prominent Golgi complexes, and rough ER. The centrosome is large and may be surrounded by microtubules.

Platelets (Fig. 11–14) have a plasma membrane with a heavy glycocalyx. The plasma membrane dips into the cytoplasm to become continuous with a system of canaliculi (the open canalicular system). Electron-microscopic markers such as thorium dioxide placed in the plasma have ready access to the canaliculi. Microfilaments of the actin–myosin system lie directly beneath the plasma membrane and among microtubules. A bundle of microtubules runs as a hoop around the periphery of the platelet and probably accounts for its lenticular shape. Platelets contain a variety of membrane-bounded granules. *Dense-core granules* 0.5 to 1.5 µm in diameter, similar to a class of synaptic vesicles, contain serotonin, ADP, ATP, and calcium. *Alpha granules,* somewhat larger and more numerous, contain various substances related to blood clotting: platelet factor 4, which neutralizes heparin; factors that increase vascular permeability and are chemotactic for neutrophils, platelet fibrinogen, actin and myosin, and ADP, ATP, and ATPase. The alpha granules are lysosomal in character, moreover, because they contain many of the acid hydrolytic enzymes characteristic of lysosomes. A few staightforward lysosomes, *lambda granules,* are present as well. There are a few mitochondria. Small profiles of smooth membrane that represent the dense tubular system are present. They concentrate calcium and

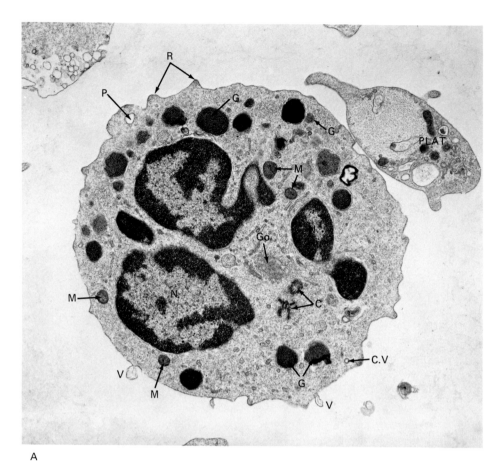

A

11–11 **A.** Electron micrograph of a normal human basophil leukocyte. This cell was taken from a person who suffered from allergic rhinitis on exposure to grass pollen, but not on exposure to ragweed pollen. When an aliquot of washed blood cells was incubated in vitro with a ragweed extract, there was no release of histamine and the basophils looked normal as shown here. The cell surface is smooth, showing only small ridges **(R)**, pockets **(P)**, and vesicular protrusions **(V)**. One platelet is adherent to the cell surface **(PLAT)**. The cytoplasm contains many typical basophilic granules **(G)**, which vary in size and shape. Also shown are the polymorphous nucleus **(N)**, four mitochondria **(M)**, the Golgi apparatus **(Go)**, the two centrioles **(C)** and a coated vesicle **(C.V)**. × 15,000. **B.** Electron micrograph of a degranulated human basophil leukocyte. This cell was taken from the same donor as that shown in part A. In

→

synthesize prostaglandins. Particles of glycogen are also present.

Cytochemistry of Blood Cells

Much may be inferred of the chemical composition of blood cells from their appearance in Romanovsky-type preparations, such as the strongly anionic nature of eosinophilic granules and the strongly cationic nature of basophilic granules. The use of selective or specific cytochemical reagents can extend this information at both the light- and electron-microscopic levels (Chap. 2). There are many chemical moieties common to many blood cells, such as ribonucleoprotein and actin. The most significant use of cytochemistry, however, has been to reveal compounds distinctive to a cell type, or to certain phases in the cycle of that cell type, or to certain subtypes; thus cytochemistry provides the basis for identifying a cell type and for understanding its function and life history.

Erythrocytes are positive for hemoglobin, gradually synthesized during their development.

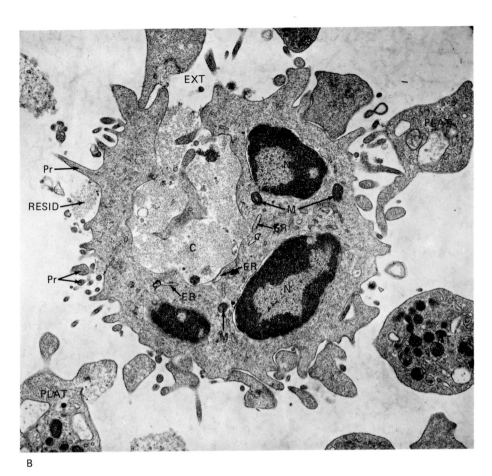

B

the same experiment, an aliquot of washed blood cells
was incubated in vitro with a grass extract. Secretion
of more than 95% of the histamine in the cells
resulted and the basophils appeared degranulated as
shown here. The cell surface is irregular, showing
numerous projections of variable appearance **(Pr)**.
Other leukocytes and platelets **(PLAT)** are adherent to
the surface of the basophil. No basophilic granules
can be seen in the cytoplasm, but a large membrane-
bounded cavity **(C)** is evident, which contains residual
granular material and communicates widely with the
exterior **(Ext)**. Further residual granular material can
be seen at the cell surface **(Resid)**. Also shown are the
polymorphous nucleus **(N)**, three mitochondria **(M)**,
and cisternae of smooth endoplasmic reticulum **(ER)**.
× 15,000. (From Hastie, R., Levy, D., and Weiss, L.
1977. J. Lab. Invest. 36:173.)

Spectrin can be localized by immunocytochemistry. The azurophilic granules of neutrophils are
lysosomal in nature because they contain lysosome-associated enzymes. The specific granules
contain a cytochemically demonstrable peroxidase. The granules of neutrophils contain many
other enzymes and metabolically active compounds (page 462), most of which can be demonstrated cytochemically. The pronounced eo-
sinophilia of the eosinophilic granule is largely
due to a major basic protein (MBP) present in the
crystalloid. This protein accounts for more than
50% of granule protein, has a molecular weight
of 11,000, and is quite rich in the amino acid arginine, which bears a strongly cationic, terminal
guanidonium group (pK > 11). The capacity of
the granules to bind eosin or other anionic dyes
seems to be due to MBP. The granules contain
lipid, reactive both with Sudan black B and with
methods for phospholipid. Myeloperoxidase is
present and can serve as a marker. Other granule
enzymes are arylsulfatase, phospholipases, acid
phosphatase, β-glucuronidase, ribonuclease, and
cathepsin. The intense metachromatic basophilia

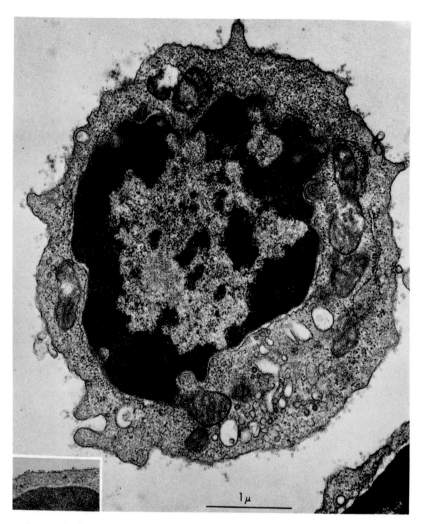

1 μ

11–12 Electron micrograph of mouse B lymphocyte.
The antibody receptors on the surface of this cell have been revealed by an antibody to the mouse antibody receptors prepared in a rabbit (rabbit antimouse immunoglobulin, RAMG). The RAMG has been linked to a large hemocyanin molecule, and this molecule, which looks like a little box under the electron microscope, serves as a label indicating the presence of the mouse antibody receptors. Note that the label is distributed rather uniformly over the surface of the B lymphocyte. This preparation was labeled at a temperature of 4° C. At this temperature the antibody receptors, which are mobile, are fixed in their uniform distribution on the cell surface. At higher temperatures, after being linked with RAMG, the antibody receptors would move to one pole of the cell and concentrate there—a phenomenon known as *capping*. In the **inset,** at the same magnification, is a portion of another mouse B lymphocyte treated in the same way, except that ferritin, an iron-bearing compound is conjugated to the RAMG. The disposition of ferritin, visualized as dense particles, indicates the distribution of antibody receptors on the surface of the mouse B lymphocyte. (From Karnovsky, M. 1972. J. Exp. Med. 136:907.)

of the specific granules of basophils is due to heparin, a strongly anionic, sulfated mucopolysaccharide. These granules are periodic acid–Schiff-positive (Chap. 2). The staining reactions of basophilic granules are quite similar to those of mast cell granules. Monocytes contain lysosomes and therefore show reactions for acid phospha-tase and other lysosome-related enzymes. Platelets and the granulocytes can be stained for glycogen, and the dense-core granules of platelets for serotonin.

It has proved of great value to characterize molecules on the surface of blood cells because many critical cellular interactions are initiated

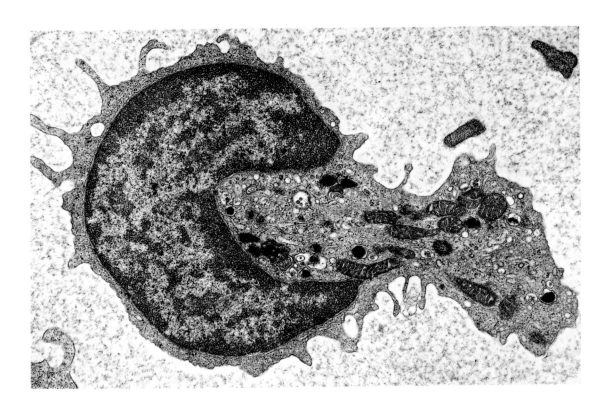

by structures there. Some of these molecules may be present in a number of cell types, as, for example, those on the surface of monocytes and some lymphocytes that bind the Fc component of antibody. Others are quite specific to a given cell type. Thus, erythrocytes have a molecule on their surface that binds transferrin, the serum protein that transports iron. This transferrin receptor permits iron to be taken up by red cells and translocated into the cell where it is used in hemoglobin synthesis. As would be expected, immature erythroid cells synthesizing hemoglobin have more of this receptor than those in which hemoglobin synthesis is complete.

On the basis of molecules on the cell surface that can be stained by immunocytochemical methods (see Chap. 2), lymphocytes may be divided into three classes: B cells, T cells, and null cells. This division, which underlies our understanding of the immune system, is discussed in the section on Lymphocytes, below.

Cytochemical data, especially from enzyme histochemistry and immunocytochemistry, are increasingly important in understanding the blood cells and hematopoietic tissues, and they will be further discussed, in this and following chapters.

11–13 Human lymphocyte. A motile lymphocyte contains a moderate number of membrane-bounded granules. Note the microvilli on the cell surface. It is likely that the lymphocyte is moving to the left, advancing with its nuclear pole. The cell assumes a hand-mirror configuration. The tail of cytoplasm has been termed a *uropod*. × 9,200. (From the work of G. A. Ackerman.)

Functions of Blood Cells

Erythrocytes

Erythrocytes transport oxygen from pulmonary alveoli to the tissues and carbon dioxide from the tissues to pulmonary alveoli. In alveoli, oxygenated blood has an oxygen tension of approximately 96 mm of Hg, whereas in systemic venous blood coming from the tissues, the oxygen tension is approximately 40 mm of Hg. Venous blood also carries carbon dioxide at a pressure of almost 50 mm of Hg, far greater than that in alveoli. As a result, oxygen diffuses through the alveolar wall into erythrocytes where it is loosely bound by the heme of hemoglobin. At the same time, carbon dioxide leaves the plasma and hemoglobin where it travels as bicarbonate and carbaminohemoglobin and diffuses into the al-

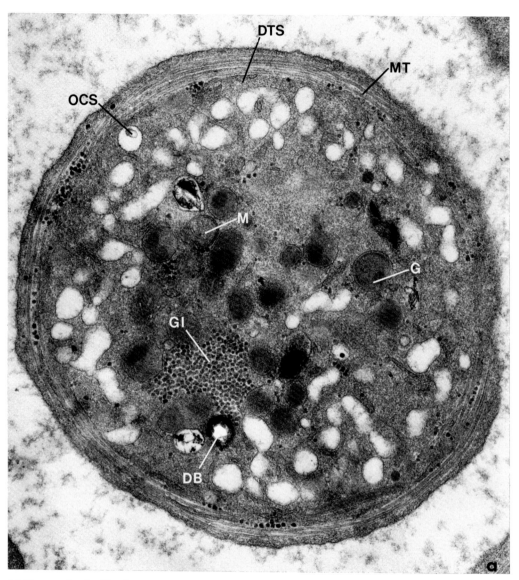

11–14 Human platelet blood. **a.** Cross section through the equatorial region of a discoid platelet. The microtubules **(MT)** form a peripheral ring. Several dense bodies **(DB)**, granules **(G)**, glycogen **(Gl)**, and mitochondria **(M)** are present. The open canalicular system **(OCS)** lies as a system of connecting tubules. In this section their surface connection is not evident, but see part a. Elements of the dense tubular system **(DTS)** are also present. × 41,000. **b.** Longitudinal section through a discoid platelet. The open canalicular system **(OCS)** lies in the center, its connection to the outside evident on the lower surface **(arrow)**. The microtubules **(MT)** are present in cross section at the poles of the platelet. Elements of the dense tubular system **(DTS)** are also present. × 41,000. (From the work of James G. White.)

veoli. When blood reaches capillaries, oxygen dissociates from the hemoglobin and diffuses through the plasma and capillary wall and out into the surrounding tissues, while carbon dioxide diffuses from the tissues into the plasma and into erythrocytes.

Hemoglobin, a globular chromoprotein of 68,000 daltons, is a tetramer, each unit consisting of a heme group associated with a polypeptide chain, the globin. The heme group is a protoporphyrin composed of four pyrrole rings coordinated through their N atom with iron.

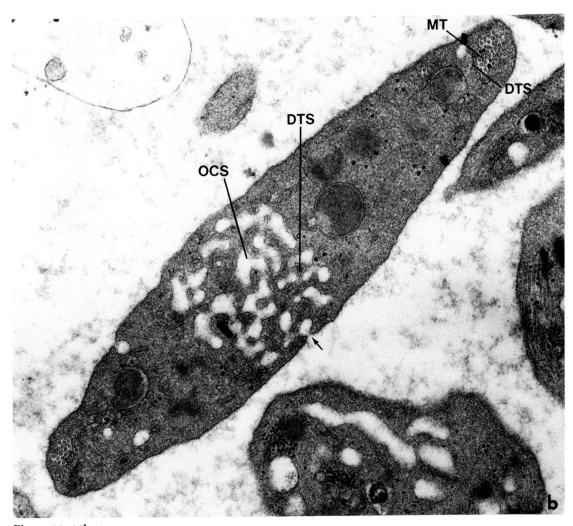

Figure 11–14b

Heme occurs not only in hemoglobin, but in myoglobin and such enzymes as catalase, peroxidase, and the cytochromes as well. Normal adult human globin consists of two alpha chains (each 241 amino acids long) and two nonalpha chains. The major adult hemoglobin, hemoglobin A (HbA) contains 2 beta chains (246 amino acids long). Each of these four chains has eight helical segments; the four chains, arranged in two pairs, are coiled in a distinctive quaternary structure into a globular molecule with the hemes lying in pockets in the center. Here the iron of heme associates with oxygen. The iron must be maintained in a ferrous form in order to transport oxygen. The oxidized form, *methemoglobin*, is inactive. Erythrocytes contain an enzyme, *methemoglobin reductase*, that maintains hemoglo-

bin in its reduced state. Hemoglobin constitutes about 33% of the weight of the cell and is in so concentrated a solution that it approaches the crystalline state. It may, in some pathological conditions, become so viscous as to reduce the plasticity of red cells and prevent efficient blood flow. The biconcave shape of erythrocytes, maintained by the subplasmalemmal framework of spectrin, efficiently makes the interior of the cell quite accessible to oxygen and carbon dioxide. In flow, the central biconcavity is commonly drawn out and the erythrocyte circulates in the shape of a cone, apex forward (Fig. 11–2). The spectrin framework also stabilizes the red cell membrane against the shearing forces encountered in flow. In spectrin-deficient animals, erythrocytes lose their biconcave shape and are short-lived. Ma-

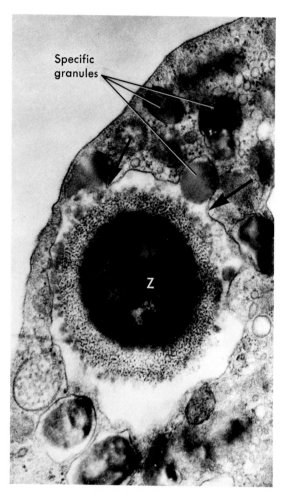

Specific
granules

Z

11–15 Phagocytic polymorphonuclear heterophil of the rabbit. This cell, harvested from the peritoneal cavity, has ingested zymosan particles **(Z)**. The specific granules of the heterophil discharge their content of hydrolytic enzymes into the phagocytic vacuole. The granule moves toward the phagocytic vacuole; its membrane fuses with the membrane of the vacuole **(arrows)**; and the contents of the granule enter the phagocytic vacuole. × 30,000. (Courtesy of D. Zucker-Franklin.)

ture erythrocytes, lacking nucleus, ribosomes, and mitochondria, have lost their capacities for protein synthesis and aerobic metabolism. They depend on glycolysis for energy, most of which is used to maintain hemoglobin in the reduced state and to maintain the internal ion concentration through active transport of ions across their semipermeable plasma membrane. Mature erythrocytes have lost the capacity to synthesize new cell membrane. They have even lost the capacity to control fully the chemical composition of their

plasma membrane. For example, the cholesterol concentration in the red cell membrane is determined by the cholesterol concentration in the plasma and not by the metabolism of the red cell. This is important because membrane plasticity, which is necessary for red cell survival, is affected by the cholesterol content of the membrane.

Neutrophils

Antimicrobial Actions. Neutrophils phagocytize and often kill bacteria and other infectious organisms that enter the body. Neutrophils are necessary to life: an individual without them or with impaired neutrophils dies of infection. A neutrophil moves toward bacteria because they release an attractant that diffuses into the surrounding tissue and interacts with the leukocyte membrane (chemotropism). There are also host factors, such as *complement* released in an inflammatory response, that attract neutrophils. The phagocytic system of neutrophils, eosinophils, and basophils has been called the *microphage system* to distinguish it from the *macrophage system* (Chap. 4). Phagocytosis is facilitated by a surface against which the microorganisms can be pinioned: bacteria suspended in a fluid-filled body cavity may escape. Phagocytosis may be enhanced by certain antibodies called *opsonins*, which neutrophils can bind to their surface.

Phagocytosis by neutrophils and other granulocytes is associated with the fusion of granules and phagosomes (Fig. 11–15, and Chap. 4). In neutrophils the specific granules usually fuse first with the phagosome, often within 30 sec of its formation. Later the azurophilic granules may combine with the phagosome. Phagocytosis requires energy and causes increased oxygen consumption.

Because they are lysosomal in character, azurophilic granules contain acid hydrolytic enzymes. They also contain *lysozyme*, an enzyme complex that hydrolyzes glycosides in the cell wall of bacteria, and a myeloperoxidase that complexes with H_2O_2 producing activated oxygen, which is bacteriocidal. Specific granules also contain lysozyme, as well as *lactoferrin*, a protein that binds ferric iron. Lactoferrin is bacteriostatic as bacteria require iron, which is unavailable when bound to lactoferrin. Lactoferrin also inhibits the production of neutrophils. This property is the basis of a feedback loop in neutrophil production: as more neutrophils are produced, more lactoferrin is produced, and thereby more inhibition is exerted on neutrophil production. Specific granules also contain cationic compounds rich in arginine and lysine, which are bacteriocidal. These granules, moreover, can generate iodides, chlorides, fatty acids, and lecithins, all of which inhibit or kill microorganisms.

Because many of the functions of neutrophils and other leukocytes are revealed in the phenomenom of inflammation, we shall next consider certain phases of inflammation. If chemical irritants or bacteria or other foreign substances penetrate the body, a series of reactions is initiated that constitutes inflammation. Inflammation is largely a phenomenon of vascular and connective tissues. The ground substance is depolymerized and becomes much less viscous. Capillaries and venules supplying the affected area become dilated, increasing its blood supply and hence its temperature. The permeability of the vascular wall is increased and plasma pours into the surrounding connective tissues, causing swelling and increased pressure on nerve endings. Cells in the locale respond. Mast cells degranulate, further intensifying inflammation. The macrophages may become hypertrophied or "activated." Circulating polymorphonuclear leukocytes, monocytes, and lymphocytes escape from capillary and postcapillary vessels and move into the site. Bacteria are phagocytized. Lymphocytes, as discussed below, may release factors called *lymphokines* with far-reaching effects on other cells and on the inflammatory process. Monocytes are transformed into macrophages and they and other cells may release kines similar to lymphokines (termed *monokines* and *cytokines*). Neutrophils, eosinophils, basophils, and macrophages may degranulate and release a large variety of substances with microcidal inflammatory and diverse further effects, as discussed under each of these cell types. Immune reactions may supervene, augmenting the population and activities of macrophages, lymphocytes, plasma cells, mast cells, eosinophils, and related cell types.

Systems of factors that are derived largely from blood plasma and consist of polypeptides and proteins, many of which are enzymes, are complexly interrelated in inflammation, blood coagulation, and immunity. The *complement system* consists of at least 10 plasma components that, when activated, react sequentially with multifold consequences. Components of complement, in conjunction with certain antibodies,

cause cell lysis. Other components induce the release of histamine from mast cells and basophils (see below), are chemotactic for neutrophils, enhance phagocytosis, induce smooth muscle contraction, and can initiate the coagulation of blood. The *kinins*, another plasma system, include compounds such as the *kallikreins* that are chemotactic for neutrophils and that induce activation of the *Hageman factor*. This factor is a plasma globulin that can convert prekallikreins to their active form and it is also both able to initiate blood coagulation and to induce lysis of the blood clot (*fibrinolysis*). One product of the kinin system is the nonapepetide *bradykinin*, which is as potent as histamine in inducing increased capillary permeability and the contraction of vascular and other smooth muscle. This system is also tied to the coagulation of blood. Other humoral substances, *prostaglandins*, have inflammatory effects, such as inducing pain, fever, and muscular contraction. The efficiency of acetylsalicylic acid (aspirin) depends on its antagonism to prostaglandins.

The ancients recognized these characteristics of inflammation: *tumor, rubor, dolor,* and *calor.* They constitute the cardinal clinical features of the acute inflammation. Leukocytes, largely neutrophils, are the preponderant cells in the immediate or acute phase of inflammation. They die after a short time. Dead and dying leukocytes mixed with serum and tissue fluids, yellow in color and creamy in consistency, are called *pus.* The activity of leukocytes underlies the swelling, redness, pain, and heat of a boil. As the acute phase of inflammation subsides and the process becomes subacute and chronic, the production and accumulation of neutrophils diminishes and macrophages come into the affected zone in larger numbers. They clear away cellular remnants and persisting irritants by phagocytosis and by releasing lytic enzymes. Most macrophages in inflammation come from circulating monocytes that leave blood vessels, move to the site of inflammation, and, as they do, are transformed into macrophages. Macrophages may in some instances accumulate and undergo further transformation into epithelioid cells and multinucleate giant cells. Indeed, the *granulomatous diseases*, which include tuberculosis and brucellosis, are characterized by nodular accumulations of macrophages and related cells.

Inflammation represents a major mechanism for controlling infectious disease, tumors, and other derangements. Inflammation is regulated by many feedback loops (for example, that of lactoferrin), but the process can escape control, become exaggerated, and can damage or kill the host. Further information related to inflammation is presented in the subsequent sections on basophils, eosinophils, and lymphocytes, and in the chapters on the connective tissues, bone marrow, thymus, lymph nodes, and spleen.

Basophils

Basophils are phagocytic motile granulocytes. Because their granules contain hydrolytic enzymes and form heterolysosomes, they undoubtedly share phagocytic-related antimicrobial features with neutrophils. Basophilic granules and those of mast cells are similar morphologically and physiologically.

Basophil granules contain heparin and histamine. Heparin is a sulfated mucopolysaccharide responsible for the metachromasia of the granules. It is an anticoagulant of blood and disperses lipid. Histamine, formed by the decarboxylation of the amino acid histidine; serotonin, which occurs in rodent basophil granules; and slow reacting substance (SRS) are vasodilating agents that induce increased vascular permeability. Unlike histamine, whose effects are prompt and transient, SRS acts in a more sustained fashion after a latent period. Slow reacting substance is lipid, possibly related to the prostaglandins. Thus the granules of basophils (and of mast cells) contain powerful mediators that affect blood vessels and intensify inflammation.

Basophils may degranulate in response to a variety of stimuli and can be important in general inflammation. However, a specific antibody-induced type of degranulation does occur. Certain antigens induce plasma cells to produce a distinctive class of antibody, immunoglobulin E (IgE), which quickly becomes fixed to the cell surface of basophils and mast cells. Loaded with IgE, basophils and mast cells remain apparently undisturbed. However, when the antigen that stimulated the production of IgE reenters the body, it combines with the IgE bound to the cell surfaces. The cells now undergo acute degranulation, releasing histamine and other mediators (Fig. 11–11, A and B). The reaction may be localized to certain shock organs such as the skin (the so-called *Prausnitz-Küstner reagenic response*) and the lungs (as in bronchial asthma); or it may be widespread and severe, as in the anaphylactic response after a bee sting or an injection of penicillin in allergic individuals.

These reactions that depend on degranulation of basophils and mast cells occur quickly and are classified as *immediate hypersensitivity*.

Basophils are also part of the initial response in a class of immunological reactions that take some time to develop, the so-called *delayed hypersensitivities* (see the section below on Cellular Immunity). Examples of delayed hypersensitivities that involve an initial basophil response are those associated with worm and viral infections, the allergic reaction in the skin after contact with certain chemicals (*cutaneous basophil hypersensitivity*), and that in tick infestations. In these reactions, basophils appear to induce inflammation, prepare the way for further immunological response, and, in the case of parasites, induce expulsion. In many cases where basophils occur, eosinophils are also present because basophils may release at least six factors chemotactic for eosinophils. These factors include eosinophilic chemotactic factor of anaphylaxis (ECF-A), tetrapeptides, and histamine. Basophils release additional substances that, on interaction with tissue factors, become chemotactic for eosinophils. Eosinophils are killer cells in certain parasitic infections. These infections induce a mast cell or basophil response that then calls in the eosinophils.

Basophils share many cytochemical and pharmacological characteristics with mast cells. However, they have a polymorphous nucleus unlike the round nucleus of mast cells. The ultrastructure of the granules of these two cell types, moreover, is similar but not the same. Some species have one cell type and not the other. Mice, for example, have mast cells and not basophils; turtles, basophils and not mast cells. Mast cells and basophils appear to have evolved as separate systems to meet similar needs and in many animals, as in human beings, supplement one another.

Eosinophils

Eosinophils, like neutrophils, are motile phagocytic granulocytes, but they lack the phagocytic capacity of neutrophils.

Eosinophils have a distinctive function: they kill the larvae of parasites that invade tissues, as in schistosomiasis, trichinosis, and ascariasis. In each of these diseases the level of circulating eosinophils may be driven to 90% of that of leukocytes. In experimental schistosomiasis in immune animals, a response involving mast cells and basophils occurs within about 5 min of the invasion of the parasite, and within about 15 min large numbers of eosinophils are on the scene. Within 2 h, eosinophils surround the larvae, virtually encapsulating them; degranulate on them, releasing MBP and other antilarval substances; and destroy them. If the eosinophil response is aborted, as can be done by administering an antieosinophilic antiserum, the parasitic invasion goes unchecked. The ability of the eosinophils to kill requires a specific antiparasitic antibody of the IgG type. In nonimmune animals (lacking an antiparasite antibody) the parasite may cause severe disease before immunity develops. Components of the host's complement systems can augment the eosinophils' antiparasite role. The parasitic larvae directly attract complement to their surface and thereby become chemotactic for eosinophils.

Basophils (and mast cells) summon eosinophils not only in parasitic infections where the eosinophil is a killer cell but in nonparasitic inflammation where the role of the eosinophil is less clear. Eosinophils do possess certain antiinflammatory capacities and can degrade inflammatory mediators released by basophils. For example, eosinophils can inactivate histamine because they contain the enzyme *histaminase*. However, the antibasophil role of the eosinophil must remain in doubt because in vitro assays show that the capacity of basophils to excite inflammation far exceeds the capacity of eosinophils to dampen it.

Lymphocytes are also important in eosinophil functions. Some of the lymphokines produced by lymphocytes in immune responses are chemotactic for eosinophils. Thus in inflammatory reactions where immune mechanisms are also activated, as in parasitic infections, both basophils (and mast cells) and lymphocytes elaborate factors chemotactic for eosinophils, bringing them to the site of reaction. Further, the increased production of eosinophils that occurs in the course of parasitic infection requires that a thymic-produced lymphocyte (T cell) serve as a helper cell (Chap. 15).

Lymphocytes

Lymphocytes are the central cell types of the immune system. The three types of lymphocytes (T cells, B cells, and null cells) look alike both with the Romanovsky stains and by conventional transmission electron microscopy, but they can be distinguished by cytochemical markers. B cells are the precursors of plasma cells, the cells that produce humoral or circulating antibody. These cells can be recognized microscopically by cytochemical demonstration of antibody molecules that cover their surface. T cells, comprising several subtypes, have both a primary role in cellular immunity and a role in the regulation of hematopoiesis, including control of the differentiation of B cells into plasma cells. T cells can be identified by distinctive marker molecules on their surface and in their interior. Null cells are lymphocytes that lack T- or B-cell markers. As expected, they represent a variegated group of cells including lymphocyte killer cells and hematopoietic stem cells. In order to understand the biology of lymphocytes and of the tissues— bone marrow–thymus, spleen, lymph nodes—of which they are an intrinsic part, a knowledge of immunity is necessary.

Immunity. The idea of immunity is rooted in infectious disease. If an individual survives an infection, he may thereafter be resistant or immune to disease caused by the infecting organism. Implicit in this phenomenon are both specificity (for the individual is resistant to the microorganism he has survived and not to others) and memory (because the immunity is long-lasting, or remembered). The immune system is a means of recognizing genetic relatedness. Thus, an individual will mount an immune response against foreign tissue but not against his own or genetically identical tissue. The immune system recognizes even slight differences between what is native to an individual and what is foreign, what is "self" and what is "nonself," and reacts against nonself. An intriguing speculation is that some forms of cancer represent a mutation that the host's immune system recognizes as nonself and therefore reacts against. The development of cancer may thus represent a failure of the immune system. Indeed, when an individual's immune system is suppressed by x rays or other means, the incidence of cancer is greatly increased. However, the immune system may in some cases lose the ability to distinguish between self and nonself and attack the host's own tissues. The process results in *autoimmune disease*. There are many such diseases of which certain thyroid, kidney, and connective tissue diseases and hemolytic anemias are examples.

The two major types of immunity are humoral immunity and cellular immunity.

HUMORAL IMMUNITY. Humoral immunity tends to be elicited by invading microorganisms that live outside of host cells and by toxins released by such microorganisms. The basis of humoral immunity is the secretion of antibody by plasma cells and by B lymphocytes undergoing transformation into plasma cells. The antibody diffuses through the blood plasma, lymph, and other fluids of the body. The large-scale secretion of antibody is triggered by antigen, and the presence of antibody throughout the fluids of the body constitutes a protective presence that eliminates or limits antigen. Antigens are particulate or colloidal substances, typically foreign to the host, which may be immunogenic (that is, capable of inducing an immune response). The surface of an invading microorganism, for example, bears many descrete antigens or *antigenic determinants*. Antibodies are proteins, for the most part gamma globulins. They are classified as immunoglobulins (Ig) and are of several types. Immunoglobulin M is a large pentameric molecule (molecular weight approximately 1,000,000) and is typically, in human beings and many animals, the first produced in an immune response. It is too large to cross the placenta and other vascular barriers. As an immune response proceeds, IgM production wanes and it is succeeded by IgG, a smaller (molecular weight approximately 160,000), more efficient, higher-affinity antibody capable of crossing the placenta (Fig. 11–16). Immunoglobulin G accounts for most of the antibodies in plasma. In secondary responses (that is, in responses occurring after reintroduction of antigen) IgG is the immunoglobulin produced. Immunoglobulin A is a secretory immunoglobulin produced in the mucosa of the respiratory tract, the gut, the genitourinary tract, mammary glands, and other places where a mucous membrane separates the body from the environment. It is produced by plasma cells beneath the epithelium and then passes through the epithelium, which secretes it into the lumen of the viscus. As it passes through the epithelium, two molecules of IgA are "dimerized" by a protein *secretory piece*, synthesized, and added by the epithelial cells of the mucosa. This dimerization may make the antibody more resistant to breakdown. Immunoglobin E is the class of immunoglobulin called *homocytotrophic*; that is, it becomes affixed to the surface of mast cells and basophils. Immunoglobin D, together with monomeric IgM, serves as receptor antibody on the surface of B lymphocytes. Its further roles have

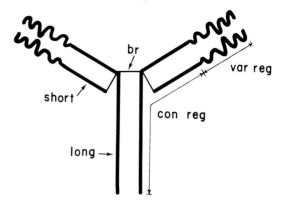

11–16 Schema of an antibody molecule of the immunoglobulin G (IgG) class. Paired long chains **(long)** diverge at the disulfide bridge **(br)**, which joins them. At the site of divergence each long chain is joined to a short chain **(short)** by a disulfide bridge. Each long chain and each short chain has a variable region **(var reg)** and a constant region **(con reg)** that lie in register. The constant region, like the handle of a key, is the same—has the same amino acid sequence—for each class of immunoglobulin. The variable region, like the part of the key inserted into the lock, is different—has a different amino acid sequence—for different antigens. The variable region of the long and short chains lying in register is that part of the antibody molecule that engages the antigen, and has been referred to as the **fab** fragment of the molecule. Because this antibody molecule possesses two fab fragments, it is divalent, that is, capable of combining with two molecules of antigen. The constant region consists of paired portions of the long chains (below the bridge) and paired portions of long chain and short chain (beyond the bridge). The constant portion of the antibody molecule, referred to as the **fc** fragment, can combine with such substrates as complement or the cell surface of macrophages, and thereby confers certain distinctive biological properties upon its antibody class.

not been well defined. Humoral immunity may be transferred from an immune to a nonimmune animal by transferring either serum (which contains antibody) or antibody-producing cells.

Plasma cells are, in essence, unicellular glands that secrete antibody. They contain the organelles associated with the synthesis and secretion of protein, namely, nucleoli, rough ER, Golgi complexes, and the secretory vesicles. They are free cells, concentrated in lymphatic tissues (lymph nodes and spleen) but found in connective tissues throughout the body. They are ovoid, measuring 10 to 20 μm in diameter.

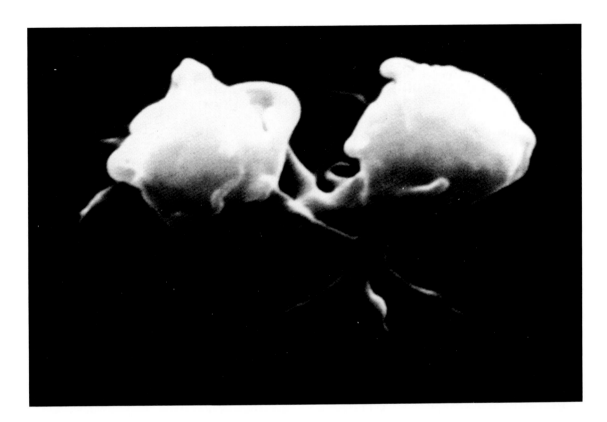

Plasma cells vary in appearance depending on phases in their life cycle (Fig. 12–17). Their distinguishing feature is the presence of antibody, which can be stained by immunocytochemical techniques, in cisternae of ER and perinuclear membranes. The Golgi apparatus of plasma cells is large. It "packages" the antibody and synthesizes and affixes a carbohydrate moiety to it. After the antibody is packaged in membrane, it travels to the cell surface in secretory vesicles and is released. The nucleus tends to lie eccentrically in the cell, displaced by the large cytocentrum. Its heterochromatin is often arranged in a pattern resembling the spokes of a wheel.

The precursors of plasma cells are B lymphocytes or, simply, B cells, which circulate in the blood (accounting for as few as 5–10% of the lymphocytes there) and also lie in characteristic loci in spleen, lymph nodes, and other lymphatic tissues. B cells can be recognized by immunocytochemical methods, which reveal molecules of immunoglobulin (types IgM and IgD) covering their surface. The antibodies lie in the plasma membrane of these B cells and readily move about in the plane of the membrane, with their antigen-combining sites directed outward and

11–17 Scanning electron micrograph of transformed platelets, displaying pseudopodia. × 30,000. (From the work of James G. White.)

free to react. These antibody molecules act as receptors for antigen. Each of the molecules of antibodies on the surface of a B cell, whether IgM or IgD, has the same antigen specificity. This specificity is very restricted, and in practice the antibody on a given B cell is capable of binding to only a single antigen. It is this narrowly focused capacity to combine with specific antigen that confers specificity on B cells and on the humoral immune system.

B lymphocytes function as follows: An antigen enters the body and, via lymph or blood, reaches sites of B-cell concentration (Chaps. 13 and 14). In these sites the antigen will "find" or "select" those B cells whose surface antibodies fit determinants on the surface of the antigen. The antigen will then link to immunoglobulin molecules on the cell surface. These antigen–antibody surface complexes now move to one pole of the B cell, at the uropod (Figs. 11–12 and 11–13) and are then taken up by endocytosis. Thus the production of plasma cells is initiated. It is a phenomenom associated with two concomitant processes. One process is the differentiation of B cells into plasma cells with concomitant high-level secretion of antibody. Curiously, those cells intermediate between B cells and the definitive small plasma cells, the *transitional cells,* produce the greatest amount of antibody. They have the appearance of large, activated lymphocytes or young plasma cells. The other process is proliferation of B cells, resulting in a B-cell clone. Indeed, it is a portion of this B-cell clone that differentiates into the plasma cells. However, a portion remains as B cells, thereby increasing the population of B cells with a given antigenic specificity. This larger pool of B lymphocytes provides the immunological memory of humoral immunity and is the basis of the heightened, brisker, and more sustained antibody response when the antigen is reintroduced, *the secondary response.* B lymphocytes may be long-lived cells, surviving months and even years. Plasma cells, on the other hand, live only about 2 weeks. Humoral immunity is an efficient process because clusters of antibody-producing cells in strategic locations produce prodigious amounts of antibodies, which, diffused through the fluids of the body, provide protection against the antigen that stimulated their production.

Some antigens, particularly those having polymeric or repeating structure, can directly induce B cells to convert into plasma cells. Most antigens cannot do this without the help of T lymphocytes. The sequence is this: a T cell recognizes and combines with antigen by means of receptors on its surface; the T cell then moves to an appropriate B cell, perhaps with the help of a macrophage (see below), and presents the antigen to the immunoglobulin receptors of the B cell.[3] Alternatively, the T cell may release lymphokines, which affect B cells. T cells may also inhibit antibody formation. Those T cells that help to convert B cells into plasma cells are a subclass, *T helper cells* (T_H). T cells that suppress the conversion are another subclass, T suppressor cells (T_S).

Macrophages are important in antibody formation. They have multiple roles in immunity but they do not have the narrow antigenic specificity of lymphocytes. As a rule, only antigens that are processed by macrophages are immunogenic. When sheep erythrocytes are injected into mice and elicit an immune response, they must be broken up into colloidal or small-sized particles. Macrophages do this. In addition, macrophages may hold antigen on their surface for long periods and present it to lymphocytes.

There is now recognized a class of cells, *antigen-presenting cells,* that includes stromal cells in lymphatic tissues, the *follicular dendritic cells* and the *interdigitating cells,* and the *Langerhans cells* of the epidermis. Their roles, and that of macrophages—which have long been accorded the function of antigen presentation—are being sorted out. These cells hold Ag on their surface, probably by cell surface receptors that bind the fc portion of the Ab molecule (fc receptors) and present the Ag to the immunocompetent lymphocytes. Without antigen-presenting cells, it is believed that many antigens would fail to reach the immunocompetent lymphocytes and that immunity would therefore fail to develop.

Macrophages destroy excess antigen. Antigen in very high (or very low) concentration causes the immune system to be unresponsive—a type of immune paralysis or *tolerance.* By phagocytizing a portion of antigen and destroying it or isolating it from immunocompetent cells, macrophages may bring the level of antigen to immunogenic levels.

Humoral antibody forms complexes with the antigen that stimulated its production and these Ag-Ab complexes will initiate a variety of responses (such as phagocytosis, lysis, activation of the complement and kinin systems, and inflammation) that tend to limit and eliminate antigen. The protective functions of the immune system are thereby accomplished.

MONOCLONAL ANTIBODIES. The immunoglobulin molecules that serve as receptors on B lymphocytes are capable, as are all antibodies, of combining quite selectively with complementary molecular conformations or *antigenic determinants* on the surface of antigens. Such complex antigens as foreign erythrocytes, viruses, bacteria, and even proteins, present many antigenic determinants on their surface. Any given B lymphocyte characteristically responds to only one antigenic determinant by producing immunoglobin molecules whose antigen-combining groups are identical (of the same *idiotype*). Therefore, as many B lymphocytes may participate in an antibody response as there are antigenic determinants on the surface of the antigen. Further, more than one B

---

[3]To become activated, a T cell must have two cell-surface receptors satisfied, as discussed below under Cellular Immunity. One of these receptors is a receptor for "self," which the macrophage as an accessory cell may satisfy.

lymphocyte may be activated by a single antigenic determinant, the idiotype produced by one lymphocyte fitting the antigenic determinant to greater or lesser degree than that produced by another—that is, with greater or lesser *affinity*. Because each lymphocyte and its clone (the lymphocytes and plasma cells derived from it by proliferation and differentiation) produce antibody molecules (of the same idiotype), this immune response is *monoclonal*. But, since an antigen bears many antigenic determinants, many different monoclonal lymphocytes are elicited in an immune response. The response is therefore *polyclonal*. If one isolates a single lymphocyte in an antibody response, it is difficult to obtain any useful amount of monoclonal antibody because the lymphocyte does not produce much antibody and does not live very long. Until recently, therefore, it has been possible to obtain monoclonal antibody in significant quantities only in unusual situations. The disease *multiple myeloma* is one such situation: A B lymphocyte differentiates into a malignant plasma cell, the *myeloma cell*, and proliferates intensely. This single malignant clone expands to completely fill the bone marrow, crowding out—with lethal consequences—all of the other hematopoietic cells and in the process producing large amounts of monoclonal antibody. Although myeloma antibody is not stimulated by a known antigen and it is abnormal, much fundamental knowledge of antibody has been learned from it.

Recently it has become possible, by an extraordinarily clever and remarkably simple means, to produce in large amount monoclonal antibody to known antigenic determinants. A single B lymphocyte obtained by micropipetting minced spleen from an animal undergoing an antibody response is fused with a myeloma cell taken from a standard laboratory strain of myeloma cells which has lost its capacity to produce antibody but which maintains its capacity for unlimited proliferation. The result of this fusion is a hybrid cell that partakes of the myeloma's capacity for unlimited proliferation—*immortality*—and of the lymphocyte's capacity for monoclonal antibody production. The hybrid cell produces much more antibody than that of the starting B lymphocyte, perhaps because the myeloma cell confers not only immortality but a heightened capacity for protein synthesis on the hybrid. Cell fusion technology can regularly be done by exposing cells to propylene glycol. The clones or *hybridomas* thus produced are the source of wholesale quantities of monoclonal antibodies.

They may be maintained in tissue culture or transplanted to the peritoneal cavity of a mouse where they form an ascites tumor producing prodigious amounts of monoclonal antibody.

Because each of the different lymphocyte idiotypes contributing to an immune response may be hybridized to a myeloma cell, one may obtain that array of monoclonal antibodies that reflects the array of antigenic determinants in the antigen. Antigens can thereby be "fingerprinted." For example, otherwise identical strains of poliomyelitis virus in an outbreak of polio may be differentiated and epidemiological studies carried out. Cell types, and subtypes, as varieties of lymphocytes or macrophages and their developmental and functional state, may be distinguished by distinctive varieties and patterns of cell surface antigens. Monoclonal antibodies prepared against antigenic determinants in such significant biological entities as the plasma membrane may be isolated and conjugated to a horseradish peroxidase or other cytochemical markers (see Chap. 2 on cytochemical methods) and an arsenal of powerful cytochemical reagents thereby created. This topic is presented more fully in the discussion in Chap. 14 of major histocompatability complex (MHC)–determined cell surface antigens on the plasma membranes of the epithelial cells of the thymus.

Monoclonal antibodies are becoming valuable in the clinic. If monoclonal antibodies are prepared against antigenic determinants that are distinctive to a tumor, the presence of that tumor and its metastases can be demonstrated by administering to the patient monoclonal antibodies tagged with radioactive isotopes. The distribution of the isotope, and inferentially of the tumor, can then be determined by scanning the whole body by using newer imaging techniques, as computer assisted axial tomography (CAT scanning) and nuclear magnetic resonance (NMR) imaging. Therapeutic use of monoclonal antibodies against tumors (immunotherapy) may be possible by conjugating a tumoricidal agent to the antibodies, which would deliver the agent specifically and in high concentration to the tumor.

CELLULAR IMMUNITY. In contrast to humoral immunity, which by the dispersion of antibody molecules has systemic scope, *cellular immunity* depends on immunologically competent cells working over short range in restricted sites where antigen is lodged. Cellular immunity is elicited by microorganisms (certain bacteria, protozoa, fungi, and viruses) that do not lie free in the host but lie intracellularly within macrophages and other cells, by diffusible products elaborated by these microorganisms, by grafts of tissue, by tumors, and by certain compounds applied to skin and other surfaces (contact hypersensitivity). In each of these varieties of cellular immunity the manifestations of the response to antigen by an immune or sensitized individual are not immediate, as they are in humoral immunity (see discussion of Arthus reaction, below), but delayed several hours. For this reason the term *delayed hypersensitivity* has been applied to cellular immunity, particularly to that variety elicited by products of the microorganisms causing cellular immunity.

Cellular immunity depends on T cells. T cells account for about 80–90% of the lymphocytes circulating in the blood and in thoracic duct lymph. They have surface receptors that are as specific for antigen as the immunoglobulin receptors of B cells. The molecular nature of the T-cell receptor for antigen is not known. However, there are functional immune response (ir) genes in T lymphocytes[4] and it is suspected that a low-molecular-weight compound with antigen-specific receptors may be coded by these genes, produced in the cell, and may move to the cell surface to serve as the antigen receptors of the T cell. T cells bear another receptor coded by the same gene complex. This receptor expresses "self." For a T cell to be activated, each of these receptors must be satisfied. In addition to presenting the Ag to the T cell, satisfying the T cell's Ag receptors, macrophages present their own surface molecules to satisfy the T cell's "self" receptors. Other distinctive substances can be demonstrated on the surface of T cells. Although the function of these substances is not known, they serve as markers. Antibodies—nowadays often monoclonal antibodies—to these substances may be prepared and, when suitably labeled, are the basis of immunocytochemical tests to detect T cells (Figs. 15–19 and 16–22). Because they may be recognized by antibody-conjugated reagents, these surface molecules are often termed *cell surface antigens.*

The cell surface antigens on T cells vary in kind and in concentration with the development of the T cell in bone marrow, thymus, and spleen

(Chap. 12). Among the antigens that mark the surface of mouse T cells are varieties of the H-2 antigens. Certain H-2 Ag also occur on the surface of many other cells and seem to be responsible for exciting the host's cellular immune response to a graft, leading to rejection of the graft. The TL or thymic leukemia antigen is a cluster of several antigens on the surface of T cells during their thymic phase of development. These antigens are not present on T cells of every strain of mouse but do appear when leukemia develops. Mouse leukemia is virally induced, so that this surface antigen may well represent the product of a viral genome integrated into a mouse chromosome. *GIX* is another such antigen. It represents a glycoprotein component of the envelope of a mouse leukemia virus and is present in the thymic phase of T-cell differentiation but not in fully differentiated T cells. One of the first discovered of the T-cell surface markers in the mouse is the Θ antigen (also termed Thy-1). It is in both immature and mature T cells, but in somewhat lesser amount in the mature cell. This antigen is also present on certain brain cells, fibroblasts, and epithelia. The Ly-1 and Ly-2,3 antigens and surface markers are found on mature T cells in mice, human beings, and other species and are valuable because they correlate with T-cell function: the Ly-1 marks T_H cells and the Ly-2,3, marks both T_s cells and T cells that kill target cells bearing a specific antigen (T_c).[5] The markers so far discussed lie on the cell surface. Other markers of T cells may be internal, such as the nuclear enzyme *terminal deoxynucleotydl transferase (Tdt)*, an enzyme distinctive to thymic T cells. This enzyme adds nucleotides to segments of DNA and may play a role in inducing T-cell mutation and immunological diversity. Another internal enzyme that marks the adult T cells of many species is an α-*naphthyl-acid esterase* located in lysosomes. Some efforts have been made to differentiate T cells from other lymphocytes morphologically, i.e., by the presence of a smooth microvillus-free surface or by nuclear shape; but these "easy methods" have proved unreliable and we are left with having to use specialized immunocytochemical and enzyme cytochemical techniques to demonstrate the markers described above.

Cellular immunity depends on the specific interaction of antigen and T cell, often at the site

---

[4]These genes are part of an extensive gene complex, a "supergene," known as the *major histocompatability complex (MHC)* a name derived from transplantation immunology (page 524). In the mouse the MHC is known as the H-2 complex and is in chromosome 17. In human beings it is termed the HL complex and lies in chromosome $\bar{6}$.

---

[5]B cells possess an Ly-4 surface antigen.

of antigen, as in the bed or vasculature of a skin graft undergoing rejection. The antigen, somewhat denatured or altered, is held on the surface of antigen presenting cells and thus presented to T cells. Again, as in B-cell stimulation, the antigen must "select" the appropriate T cell. The stimulated T cell then undergoes clonal expansion and a portion of that clone probably engages in the cellular immune response, i.e. the production of lymphokines. The remaining cells of the clone constitute a bank of memory cells. Clonal selection, memory, and specificity are inherent in the phenomenon of cellular immunity, parallel to the B-cell response in humoral immunity. The fate of the activated lymphokine-producing T cells is unknown. They may die or become part of the memory pool.

Lymphokines have been identified on the basis of biological activity. Almost one hundred types have been postulated! Most probably, when they are chemically characterized, single lymphokines will be found to have multiple activities and, therefore, the total number of lymphokines will be considerably reduced. As the biology of lymphokines is further studied it is becoming evident that monocytes and macrophages can produce similar factors (hence, the term *monokine*), as can other cell types (hence, the term *cytokine*). Quite possibly, these small nonimmunoglobulin molecules represent a general way by which cells may affect one another. Lymphocytes, of course, are distinctive because their lymphokine production can be specifically activated by antigen.

The actions of lymphokines may be appreciated in an example of cellular immunity, the rejection of a homograft of skin.[6] After such skin is grafted, T lymphocytes (which, as discussed in Chap. 12, circulate and recirculate through the tissues) enter the bed of the graft, flowing through its blood vessels. Those T cells bearing surface receptors specific for the foreign antigen encounter and interact with that antigen held on the surface of macrophages. The antigen is often associated with blood vessels of the graft, the first foreign place the host T cell reaches at the graft site. The lymphocytes become activated and

produce and release lymphokines. One of the best characterized of the lymphokines is *macrophage migration inhibition factor* (MIF). Macrophages normally wander in and out of tissues. However, if they are exposed to MIF, they cease wandering and accumulate—in this example, in the bed of the graft. *Macrophage activation factor* (MAF), another lymphokine (perhaps overlaping MIF in activity) would activate these macrophages (see Chap. 4), making them "irate." *Lymphotoxin* (LT) damages or destroys cells other than lymphocytes. *Lymphocyte blastogenic factor* (BF) induces "blast formation" and division in lymphocytes. Other lymphokines released by the antigen-stimulated T cells are chemotactic for basophils and eosinophils and bring these granulocytes to the scene. Some lymphokines affect vascular permeability; others are generally cytotoxic. The net effect of this complex process is the rejection of the graft.

A classic type of cellular immunity serving as an example of delayed hypersensitivity occurs in tuberculosis as the *tuberculin reaction*. A purified protein derivitive (PPD) of tubercle bacilli is injected into the skin of a tuberculous animal. This animal is sensitive to many antigens in the bacilli, including PPD. The site of injection is first apparently unreactive, and then in 4 to 8 h redness and induration (hardness) appear. The reaction builds to a peak in 24 to 48 h, thus "delayed hypersensitivity," and then subsides. It may consist only of redness and some swelling, but if severe it can be painful and ulcerated. The basis of the reaction is that circulating T lymphocytes sensitive to the PPD, i.e., having surface receptors for the PPD, enter the site where tubercle bacilli lie; there they react through intermediary macrophages with the bacilli's PPD and liberate lymphokines. These lymphokines immobilize local and passing macrophages, call in lymphocytes and other cells, and induce the inflammation and cell damage characteristic of the tuberculin reaction. Despite the fact that sensitized lymphocytes initiate the process, the major cell types present and effecting the reaction are monocytes and macrophages. Thus this process, like that of the skin graft presented above, depends on sensitized lymphycytes moving to the site and acting locally.

In contrast, an example of humoral antibody-mediated immunity is the *Arthus reaction*. In this case, an antigen is injected into the skin of an individual who is immunized against that antigen and carries circulating antibody to it.

[6]A homograft is within the same species but between different strains, such as the different strains of inbred mice (AKR to C57B). An *isograft* is a graft from donor to recipient of the same strain (e.g., AKR to AKR). Because individuals of the same strain (and same sex) are the same genetically, isografts are not rejected. Humans, being outbred, may have isografts only between identical twins.

Within minutes after injection, the skin is inflamed: red, painful, hot, and hard. This reaction is initiated by injected antigen combining with circulating antibody at the site. The antigen–antibody complex combines with complement and other serum factors and causes local injury, inducing inflammation and an accumulation of large numbers of neutrophils.

In summary, lymphocytes are central in the immune response. B lymphocytes are precursors to plasma cells. They synthesize antibody and underlie humoral antibody production. T lymphocytes are the basis of cellular immunity, a complex of immune reactions directed toward intracellular bacteria, viruses, protozoal parasites and fungi, tumors, tissue grafts, and certain soluble, diffusible compounds. In addition, T cells may regulate humoral antibody production. T_H lymphocytes, a subset of T cells, permit B lymphocytes to mount a humoral response; T_s lymphocytes, another subset, suppress B-cell maturation and forestall a humoral response. Because of their specificity for antigen and their capacity for establishing immunological memory (immunity), lymphocytes are called "immunologically competent cells."

THE DEVELOPMENT OF IMMUNOLOGICAL COMPETENCE. At birth most mammals are immunologically quiet, both because their immunological capacities are not fully developed and because the placental barrier has shielded them from foreign material. The newborn, moreover, is protected against many infectious diseases by maternal antibodies that cross the placental barrier and circulate in its body. Such transplacental antibody constitutes a *passive immunization*. The immunological competence of a fetus increases as the time of parturition approaches, and within a few days of birth the newborn's own immunological mechanisms become active because of exposure to antigens. That the fetus does possess increasing immunological capacity can be shown experimentally by its production of antibody after direct injection of antigen.

Lymphocyte Control of Hematopoiesis. T lymphocytes appear to play a significant role in the production of blood cells (hematopoiesis). Intact animals will generate high levels of eosinophils when infected with nematode parasites whose larvae encyst in host muscle, but athymic animals lacking T cells are unable to bring their eosinophils over basal levels. When supplied with T cells, however, animals deficient in T cells can generate high levels of eosinophils. Under certain conditions, moreover, heightened neutrophilopoiesis also seems to depend on the thymus. With regard to erythrocytes, colonies derived from cell precursors in tissue culture increase in number and size when cocultured with T cells. Certain anemias, such as the Diamond-Blackfan syndrome, may be due to T_s cells inhibiting erythropoiesis. The best known and best understood example of T-cell control of hematopoiesis concerns the differentiation of B cells into plasma cells after stimulation by antigen. T_H and T_s cells regulate this process, as described above. Thus T lymphocytes may exert a general control over hematopoiesis, of which the differentiation of B lymphocytes into plasma cells is but an example.

Monocytes

Monocytes are the precursors of macrophages. Their functions are discussed in Chap. 4.

Platelets

Platelets are essential in preventing and staunching hemorrhage. They seal off small breaks in blood vessels, they participate in blood coagulation, and they maintain the competence of endothelium. If a blood vessel is cut and its endothelial continuity broken, certain plasma proteins—notably *Von Willebrand's factor*—are absorbed upon the exposed subendothelial collagen and other extracellular connective tissues. Within seconds circulating platelets establish contact with this subendothelial tissue and adhere to it. The platelets spread out over the damaged zone and their surface becomes altered, so that newly arrived platelets adhere to them and a hemostatic *platelet plug* is formed. As circulating platelets join the plug, they change from the discoid or lenticular form to a flattened or spherical shape with spicule-like pseudopodia (Fig. 11–17). These pseudopodia undoubtedly facilitate plug formation. This *primary aggregation* of platelets is induced by a number of factors: ADP (adenosine diphosphate) released from adherent platelets, epinephrine, and the plasma protein *thrombin*. Aggregation, moreover, is dependent upon *plasma fibrinogen* and *calcium*. As the process unfolds, the adherent platelets undergo a *release reaction*, a type of secretion wherein the platelets discharge first their dense granules and then their alpha and lambda granules. Non-granular platelet substances are also released. The release reaction causes even a larger build-up of aggregated platelets, or *secondary aggregation*.

Directly after vascular injury, during platelet aggregation, *blood clotting* or *coagulation* is initiated by plasma factors and factors released from the damaged vessel. Blood coagulation is the consequence of the sequential interactions, or *cascade*, of perhaps thirteen plasma proteins. The last step in this cascade is the conversion of the monomer plasma protein *fibrinogen* to the linear polymer *fibrin* through the action of the plasma enzyme *thrombin*. Fibrin forms an interlacing network of slender fibers, running among the platelets and trapping erythrocytes and other blood cells. The result is a jelly-like bulky clot that, with the platelet plug, serves to block bleeding. Although the blood clot may be initiated without platelets, the adherent platelets are essential to the production of a useful clot. They display great procoagulant activity by which they accelerate and magnify the process of blood coagulation. The platelet surface, exposing phospholipids such as platelet factor-3 and other substances, serves to collect coagulation proteins and facilitate their cascade. Moreover, many platelet factors secreted in the release reaction promote coagulation.

A blood clot may not only block bleeding, it may also obstruct the flow of blood by bulging into the vascular lumen. Such bulging is considerably reduced by the contraction of the clot, *clot retraction*. This platelet function is accomplished by the contractile proteins actin and myosin and adenosine triphosphate (ATP) and ATPase contained in platelets. With its injury covered by the clot, the vessel heals and its endothelium is regenerated. The clot is no longer needed. A plasma protein *plasminogen* is converted to the hydrolytic enzyme *plasmin* by *plasminogen activators* secreted by endothelial cells, and plasmin dissolves the clot.

Related to their role in hemostasis, platelets maintain the competence of endothelium. When the level of circulating platelets is reduced below about 60,000/ml^3, *(thrombocytopenia)*, fine blood vessels lose their competence and blood seeps out of them *(thrombocytopenic purpura)*. Restore platelets to normal levels and vascular competence is restored.

[See Chap. 12 for References and Selected Bibliography.]

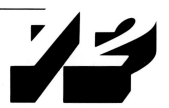

The Life Cycle of Blood Cells

Leon Weiss

Origin and Development of Blood Cells

Blood cells, like keratinocytes in skin and epithelium in gut, have a short life span. But they are constantly renewed in specialized centers, *hematopoietic tissues*, and their numbers are thereby kept constant. The system, moreover, is responsive. In infection, for example, hematopoiesis may be intensified and large numbers of leukocytes produced. Blood cells are normally released to the circulation only when sufficiently mature. They circulate within blood vessels but may temporarily stop circulating and become marginated cells. Erythrocytes and platelets remain within the vasculature. However, leukocytes will leave blood vessels and enter the perivascular tissue where they function, undergo cellular transformation, or are destroyed. Or, apparently unchanged, they may reenter the circulation, often via lymphatic vessels.

Sites of Production of Blood Cells

The major discrete hematopoietic tissues are bone marrow, spleen, lymph nodes, and thymus. There are other large concentrations of hematopoietic tissue, notably in the walls of the gastrointestinal tract. Prenatally hematopoiesis also occurs in yolk sac and liver and other sites. Except for the thymus, which has entodermal, mesenchymal and, perhaps, ectodermal components, the major hematopoietic organs in mammals are of mesenchymal origin. They contain a stroma made up of reticular cells and fibers, are supplied by vessels and nerves, and are enclosed by a capsule and trabeculae. The stroma holds free cells, including the blood cells and their precursors, macrophages, plasma cells, and mast cells.

Prenatal Hematopoiesis

Hematopoiesis in the human embryo begins in the second week of life, extraembryonically, in the wall of the yolk sac. Small nests of hematopoietic cells, largely erythroblastic (that is, producing erythrocytes), lie in mesenchyme surrounded by developing blood vessels. These foci constitute *blood islands*. The vessels enlarge and form a network within the wall of the yolk sac, connect to the systemic intraembryonic vessels through the vitelline vasculature, and become part of the circulation. By the sixth week of embryonic life erythropoietic foci appear in the liver, which becomes the major hematopoietic center. Hepatic granulocytopoiesis is minor, but there is moderate production of platelets and macrophages. Bone marrow appears in the clavicle in the second month and, with increased formation of bone, becomes extensive. It becomes the dominant hematopoietic organ in the latter half of gestation, when hematopoiesis in the liver wanes, and throughout postnatal life. All of the blood cells except T lymphocytes are produced in the marrow, and even T cells originate in marrow as stem cells and migrate to the thymus where they differentiate. From the second month of gestation the thymus engages in restricted hematopoiesis, the production of T cells.

A minor level of hematopoiesis, largely erythropoietic, becomes established in the spleen in the third fetal month and fades in the fifth. The spleen and lymph nodes receive and stock T cells from the thymus as early as the second fetal month, but only in the first postnatal weeks do the stocks become large. Although the liver is inactive hematopoietically after birth, it does retain its potential for hematopoiesis. In cases of bone marrow failure, hematopoiesis may be resumed there (and in the spleen), a phenomenon called *extramedullary hematopoiesis*.

Hematopoietic Stem Cells

A hematopoietic stem cell is capable of both sustained proliferation (producing a clone) and differentiation into mature blood cells. If only a portion of the clone differentiates into blood cells a population of stem cells is maintained. A stem cell may be multipotential, able to differentiate into any of the blood cells, or it may be of more limited potential, such as the stem cell capable of differentiating only into monocytes and neutrophils.

The existence of a pluripotential hematopoietic stem cell, which had been in doubt, has been demonstrated largely by the work of Till and McCulloch and their associates. The demonstration, although secure, is rather indirect because the stem cell has no distinguishing characteristic or marker, like, for example, the hemoglobin of red blood cells or the immunoglobulin receptor on B cells. It depends upon injecting cells that bear distinctive chromosomal markers (revealed in a metaphase karyotype) into lethally irradiated hosts, in the following type of experimental model.

After lethal irradiation (more than 900 rads) a mouse dies with all of its blood cells profoundly depleted (pancytopenia). Death may be averted if the mouse is given a suspension of living bone marrow cells from another mouse of the same inbred strain. The recipient mouse survives and in early stages of its recovery shows in both bone marrow and spleen, against a background of irradiation-induced devastation, grossly visible nodules that represent colonies of proliferating hematopoietic cells (Fig. 12–1). These colonies will grow and differentiate, and within weeks bone marrow and spleen are restored. The cellular composition of the hematopoietic colonies varies. Many of them contain only one or two types of blood cell but a significant number contain each of the blood cell types (Fig. 12–2). There is evidence that each of these colonies, including those with multiple blood cell types, is a clone (i.e., derived from a single hematopoietic cell precursor).

The evidence for such clones is obtained by irradiating the donor marrow cells severely, but not lethally, to induce chromosomal damage. This damage occurs in a widespread unpredictable way and results in cells each with uniquely or highly distinctively abnormal chromosomes (Fig. 12–3). Becker, Wu, Till, and McCulloch found that when such irradiated donor cells containing uniquely damaged chromosomes form splenic or bone marrow colonies in lethally irradiated recipients, different hematopoietic cell types within a given colony bear the same distinctive karyotype. This finding reveals that different blood cell types, such as erythrocytes, granulocytes, and monocytes, can originate from

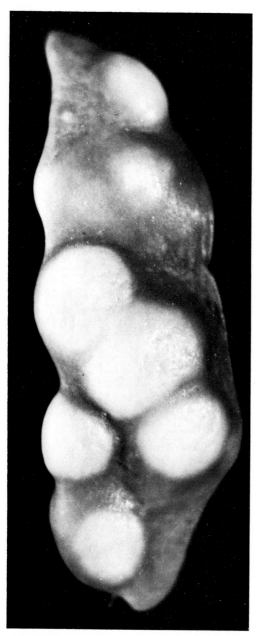

12–1 Splenic nodules. This spleen was removed
from an animal given lethal irradiation and
then a "rescuing" injection of bone marrow cells. The
stem cells, which constitute a portion of the marrow,
circulated to the irradiated spleen where they
remained, proliferated, and formed these macroscopic
colonies. Later these colonies will coalesce and the
normal structure of the spleen will be restored. (From
the work of J. Till and E. McCulloch.)

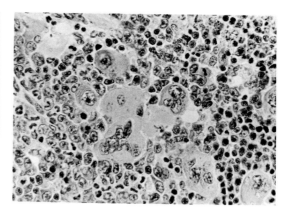

12–2 Splenic nodule. A number of splenic nodules
have a diverse hematopoietic population
including virtually all hematopoietic cell types. This
light-microscopic field is from such a nodule. (From
the work of W. T. Wu, J. Becker, J. Till, and E.
McCulloch.)

12–3 "Unique" mouse karyotype. The clonal nature
of the splenic colonies exemplified in Fig.
12–1 is revealed by distinctive or unique karyotypes
in the donor marrow cells. These karyotypes are
induced by lightly irradiating the donor cells (see
text). **Arrow** points to the distinctively damaged
chromosomes that serve as a marker. (From the work
of W. T. Wu, J. Till, and E. McCulloch.)

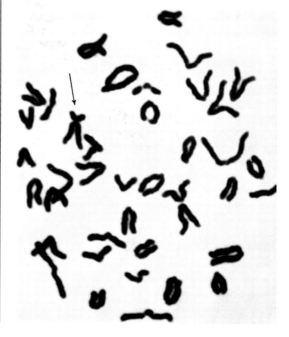

the same stem cell. Further evidence supporting the clonal nature of splenic colonies includes a linear relationship between the number of nucleated donor cells and the number of splenic and bone marrow colonies, and the resemblance of the irradiation–survival curve of colony-forming cells to that of single cells in tissue culture or tumor transplants.

The greatest concentration of multipotential stem cells in the adult, as determined by spleen colony assay, is in the bone marrow. The total number in the marrow of the mouse may be 40,000 stem cells. In contrast, the spleen may have only 2,000. The vastly greater capacity of the marrow relative to the spleen to restore an irradiated recipient is explicable by its 20-fold superiority in stem cell content. But even its relatively high content of stem cells does not represent, for the marrow, a high concentration; in the mouse it is 1 per 10,000 nucleated cells. Stem cells circulate, and there are approximately 10 in each milliliter of blood, which represents 1 per million nucleated blood cells, one-hundredth the concentration in the marrow. Stem cells circulate in the fetus and are present in fetal liver and bone marrow. When hepatic hematopoiesis declines, the number of circulating stem cells becomes unusually high, suggesting their large-scale emigration from liver to marrow.

Although no direct evidence of the structure of the multipotential hematopoietic stem cell exists, indirect evidence strongly indicates that structurally it is a lymphocyte, although many investigators eschew that term and prefer to call it a *candidate stem cell* (Figs. 12–4 and 12–21). The indirect evidence of its appearance is garnered from experiments carried out by Van Bekkum and his colleagues, using the Till and McCulloch spleen colony assay to measure the number of stem cells in a bone marrow suspension. The relative number of multipotential stem cells is greatly increased if dividing hematopoietic cells are destroyed by treating the suspension with vincristine, a drug whose action is like that of x rays.[1] The number of multipotential stem cells is further increased by subjecting the marrow suspension to density-gradient centrifu-

gation and obtaining a number of fractions, one of which can be determined to be rich in stem cells by spleen colony assay. By these methods, the stem cell concentration in a marrow suspension may be increased by a factor of 40 or more. In proportion to the increase in stem cells is the presence of a cell type, the candidate stem cell, which is lymphocytic in appearance (as seen in Fig. 12–4). Because the existence of multipotential stem cells was first clearly demonstrated on the basis of colonies in the splenic assays of Till and McCulloch, this cell has been termed the colony forming unit–spleen (CFU-S). It circulates in the blood as one of the *null cells*, one of the lymphocyte types that is neither T cell nor B cell.

The above discussion has been confined to the multipotential stem cell (CFU-S). There are stem cells derived from CFU-S capable of differentiating only into red cells or into white cell types. These more restricted stem cells, revealed by specialized tissue culture techniques, are discussed below under Culture of Erythrocyte Stem Cells and under Culture of Granulocyte and Monocyte Stem Cells.

The Life Cycle of Erythrocytes

The earliest erythroid cell recognizable in Romanovsky-stained smears of bone marrow is a fully endowed cell having nucleus, ribosomes, mitochondria, Golgi apparatus, and so forth. It serves as a stem cell for erythropoiesis, the production of erythrocytes. The nucleated precursor cells of erythrocytes are called *erythroblasts*.

In Romanovsky preparations, hemoglobin binds the anionic dye eosin because its globin is strongly cationic; RNA binds the cationic dye methylene blue$^+$ and the azures$^+$ because its phosphate groups are strongly anionic.[2] Accordingly, in early-stage erythroblasts with many ribosomes and little hemoglobin, the cytoplasm is stained deeply with basic dyes (blue in Romanovsky stains). In late stages of development, on the other hand, with few ribosomes and abundant hemoglobin, the cytoplasm is deeply stained with acid dyes (red in Romanovsky stains). Therefore, early erythroblasts are called

---

[1]Multipotential stem cells divide infrequently. They are, in fact, held in reserve and are not even in the cell cycle, being in G_0 (Chap. 1). It is left to the more differentiated stem cells to proliferate and differentiate, carrying on the normal business of the bone marrow, and these dividing cells are highly sensitive to x rays or to *radiomimetic* drugs.

[2]Positively charged dyes are termed *basic dyes* and negatively charged dyes are termed *acid* by histologists. Tissue components that bind basic dyes are called basophilic and those that bind acid dyes, acidophilic. See Chap. 2.

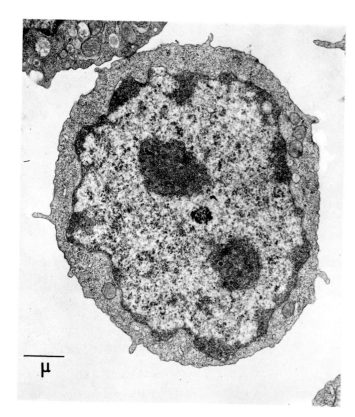

μ

12–4 Candidate stem cell. There are no obvious morphological signs indicating cellular differentiation. The cytoplasm is rich in free ribosomes. × 15,130. (From the work of Van Bekkum et al. 1971. Blood 38:547.)

basophilic erythroblasts,[3] and late erythroblasts having almost the true color of mature red cells are called orthochromatic erythroblasts. (The term normoblast is commonly applied to orthochromatic erythroblasts.) In intermediate stages, the hue of the cytoplasm represents a combination of the colors of the acid and basic dyes, and the cells are therefore termed polychromatophilic erythroblasts (Figs. 12–5 [here and color insert] to 12–7). Cell diameter decreases as erythroblasts differentiate, the basophilic erythroblast being about 15 μm in diameter, the orthochromatic erythroblasts or normoblasts, only 8 to 10 μm. The erythroblast pool is maintained by proliferation of basophilic and polychromatophilic erythroblasts. Normoblasts are postmitotic, that is, they do not divide.

By electron microscopy the cytoplasm of erythroblasts contains polyribosomes, small Golgi complexes, mitochondria, a few lysosomes, hemoglobin, ferritin, scanty endoplasmic reticulum

(ER), some microtubules, actin, and spectrin. Basophilic and early polychromatophilic erythroblasts contain abundant polyribosomes. By the orthochromatic stage, the polyribosomes are considerably reduced in both concentration and ribosomal number. The density of the cytoplasm, owing to the hemoglobin, increases throughout maturation. Ferritin, a protein able to store as many as 2,500 iron atoms, may be scattered as single molecules or in the aggregated form, hemosiderin. Hemosiderin may be collected into membrane-bound granules, siderosomes. Iron is transported by a plasma iron-binding globulin, transferrin, to transferrin receptors on the surface of erythroid cells. Here the iron flips to the inside of the cell for storage (as ferritin or hemosiderin) or for use in hemoglobin synthesis (Chap. 11). In basophilic erythroblasts a bit of rough ER is present, but even this rapidly diminishes. One or more Golgi complexes occur, and these too become quite small and disappear by the orthochromatic phase. Mitochondria diminish in number and size in polychromatophilic cells. A few remain in orthochromatic erythroblasts (normoblasts) and they are absent in mature erythrocytes (see Fig. 12–21).

---

[3]Some authors recognize a proerythroblast as less differentiated than the basophilic erythroblast. It is a similar cell but somewhat larger.

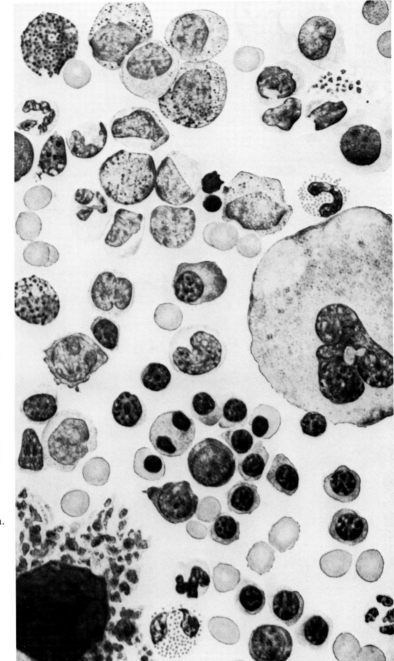

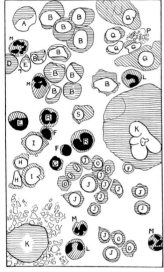

12–5 Composite plate of blood cells. See special section for color figure and lengthy caption.

With maturation, the nucleus becomes smaller, markedly heterochromatic, and nearly spherical and loses nucleoli. Just before nuclear loss, the nucleus with a thin rim of cytoplasm occupies one pole of the cell, and at the other pole is the bulk of the cytoplasm. The poles break apart and the fragment containing the nucleus is rather rapidly phagocytized. The freed anucleate pole is an erythrocyte (see following section on Reticulocytes). The thin layer of cytoplasm surrounding the discarded nucleus carries on its plasma membrane certain cell surface receptors that may

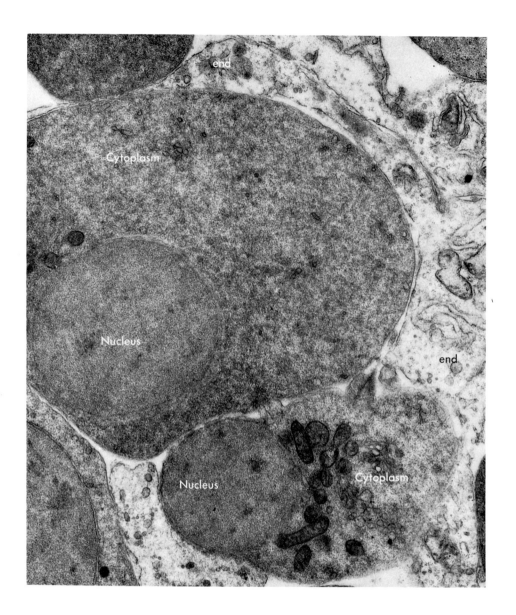

12–6 Polychromatophilic erythroblasts, bone marrow
of the rat. Two polychromatophilic
erythroblasts press against different points of the
endothelium (end) of vascular sinuses of the marrow.
The erythroblasts are markedly polarized. The
cytoplasm, at one pole, contains ribosomes and
mitochondria as well as hemoglobin. The nuclear pole
is surrounded by a thin rim of hemoglobinized
cytoplasm. The nuclear pole will be detached and
phagocytized, and the cytoplasmic pole will become a
reticulocyte. × 40,000. (From Weiss, L. 1965. J.
Morphol. 117:467.)

be useful in erythroblast maturation but not in
discarded erythrocytes. Nuclear loss regularly
occurs near the orthochromatic stage. The nucleus may be lost at earlier stages, particularly in
intensified erythropoiesis, resulting in polychromatophilic or even basophilic erythrocytes.

Reticulocytes

Freshly produced erythrocytes normally contain
some ribosomes, yet fewer than 1% have enough
to be polychromatophilic or basophilic in Ro-

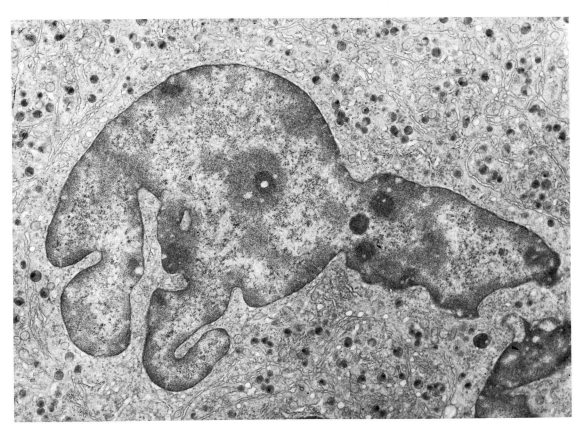

12–19 Electron micrograph of a megakaryocyte in human bone marrow. The nucleus is large and polymorphous. The cytoplasm contains granules of varying density and small mitochondria. The arresting cytoplasmic characteristic is the extensive system of demarcation membrane, which loculates platelet zones in the peripheral cytoplasm. (See Fig. 12–20.) Later the platelets will separate from the megakaryocyte and become free circulating structures. × 9,300. (From the work of I. Berman.)

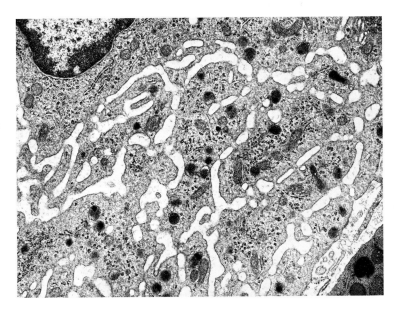

12–20 Electron micrograph of megakaryocyte in rat bone marrow. A portion of the nucleus and central cytoplasm is at the upper margin. Most of the peripheral cytoplasm is clearly demarcated into platelet zones. × 10,500.

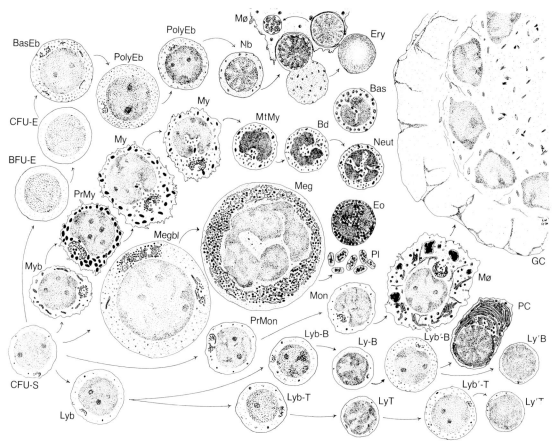

12–21 This schema shows stages in the differentiation of each of the blood cell lines as seen by electron microscopy. The multipotential stem cell (*colony forming unit–spleen*, **CFU-S**) is in the lower left corner and the various blood cell types radiate from it.

Along the topmost arc are the developing red cells. The first stages in erythrocyte differentiation are *erythroid burst forming units* (**BFU-E**) and *erythroid colony forming units* (**CFU-E**). These forms have not been seen as such; they are recognized by the colonies that derive from them in tissue culture. Their structure in this schema is, therefore, inferred. The *basophilic erythroblast* (**BasEb**) is rich in ribosomes and therefore would be deeply basophilic in Romanovsky preparations. Hemoglobin becomes evident in *polychromatophilic erythroblasts* (**PolyEb**), the early forms being relatively rich in ribosomes and poor in hemoglobin, and the later forms rich in hemoglobin and poor in ribosomes. Hemoglobin is almost fully developed and ribosomes quite depleted in *orthochromatic erythroblasts* or *normoblasts* (**Nb**). At this stage, moreover, the cells are postmitotic. Nuclear and cytoplasmic poles separate. The nuclear pole, surrounded by a rim of cytoplasm, is phagocytized by a macrophage (**Mφ**). The anucleate erythrocytes, still containing ribosomes and some

mitochondria, called *reticulocytes* after supravital staining, differentiate into a mature erythrocyte (**Ery**). Both reticulocytes and mature erythrocytes circulate.

The differentiation of neutrophilic leukocytes from the CFU-S is shown in the next arc. The first stage is the *myeloblast* (**Myb**). Then, in the *promyelocyte* (**PrMy**) primary granules appear, the nucleus begins to indent, and the cell grows larger. In the *myelocyte* stage (**My**) primary granule formation stops and secondary granule formation starts. The nucleus is increasingly indented, heterochromatic, and segmented. The metamyelocyte (**MtMy**) is smaller and postmitotic. The granule composition is definitive and the nucleus is increasingly heterochromatic and segmented. In the band form (**Bd**) and the mature neutrophil (**Neut**), nuclear segmentation is completed. An eosinophil (**Eo**) is shown below the neutrophil and a basophil (**Bas**) above.

Megakaryocyte development, presented in the third arc, depends on the development of polyploidy by endomitosis in a large mononuclear cell, a *megakaryocytoblast* (**Megbl**). Then, in its postendomitotic phase, the megakaryocyte (**Meg**) develops, undergoing cytoplasmic maturation and nuclear polymorphism. Platelets (**Pl**) are produced from the cytoplasm of megakaryocytes.

Monocytes (**Mon**), presented in the fourth

ectoplasm; it is finely granular and contains packets of microfilaments but is largely free of organelles (Figs. 12–5 [here and color insert], and 12–18 to 12–21). Megakaryocytes lie against the outside of vascular sinuses in bone marrow, delivering platelets through mural apertures directly into the vascular lumen (Figs. 12–18 and 13–4). They may deliver individual platelets or ribbons of platelets (as tickets unwinding from a spool) that subsequently separate into individual platelets in the vascular bed. Platelets are released as cytoplasmic fragments in which microtubules are present only in short segments and granules seem randomly located. Later, perhaps in the spleen, the microtubules link to form the definitive peripheral ring, the platelets assume their mature lenticular shape, and their granules lie centrally. Circulating platelets in human beings have a life span up to about 10 days. Platelets are most likely used randomly, that is, without reference to age.

There is good evidence that a humoral substance (or substances), *thrombopoietin,* stimu-

lates the maturation of megakaryocytes and the rate of platelet production. Platelet-stimulating activity is increased in the serum of individuals who have low blood platelet levels *(thrombocytopenia).* The assay for thrombopoietin depends on the uptake of radioactive selenium (as selenomethionine-75) or sulfur (as $Na_2^{35}SO_4$) by megakaryocytes and the determination of the rate at which radioactive platelets appear in blood.

References and Selected Bibliography

General

Abramson, S., Miller, R. G., and Phillips, R. A. 1977. Identification of pluripotent and restricted stem cells of the myeloid and lymphoid systems. J. Exp. Med. 145:1567.

Bloom, W., and Bartelmez, G. W. 1940. Hematopoiesis in young human embryos. Am. J. Anat. 67:21.

De Bruyn, P. P. H. 1944 and 1946. Locomotion of blood cells in tissue culture. Anat. Rec. 89:43; 95:177.

Goldstein, G. 1978. Polypeptides regulating lymphocyte differentiation. *In* Differentiation of Normal and Neoplastic Hematopoietic Cells, Clarkson, B., Marks, P. A., Till, J. E. (eds.). Cold Spring Harbor Laboratory, New York: Vol A, p. 455.

Isaacs, R. 1930. The physiological histology of bone marrow. Folia Haematol. (Leipzig) 40:395.

Jaffe, R. H. 1938. The reticuloendothelial system. *In* H. Downey (ed.), Handbook of Hematology, vol. 2. New York: Paul B. Hoeber, Inc.

Jordon, H. E. 1933. The evolution of blood-forming tissues. Q. Rev. Biol. 8:58.

Kindred, J. E. 1942. A quantitative study of the hematopoietic organs of young adult albino rats. Am. J. Anat. 71:207.

Metcalf, D., and Moore, M. A. S. 1971. Haemopoietic Cells. North-Holland Research Monographs, Front. Biol. 24. Amsterdam: North-Holland Publishing Co.

Metchnikoff, E. 1893. Lectures on the Comparative Pathology of Inflammation. Starling, F. A. and E. H. (trans.). London: Kegan Paul, Trench, Trubner and Co.

Miklem, H. S., Ford, C. E., Evans, E. P., and Gar, J. 1966. Interrelationships of myeloid and lymphoid cells: Studies with chromosome-marked cells transfused into lethally irradiated mice. Proc. R. Soc. Lond. (Biol.) 165:78.

Strominger, J. L., Ferguson, W., Fuks, A., Kaufman, J., Orr, H., Parham, P., Robb, R., Terhorst, C., Giphart, M., and Mann, D. 1978. Isolation and structure of HLA antigens. *In* Differentiation of Normal and Neoplastic Hematopoietic Cells, Clarkson, B., Marks, P. A., Till, J. E. (eds.). Cold Spring Harbor Laboratory, New York: Vol A, p. 467.

Trentin, J. J. 1970. Influence of hemopoietic organ stroma (hematopoietic inductive microenvironments) on stem cell differentiation. *In* Regulation of Hematopoiesis, vol. I, Red Cell Production, Gordon, A. S. (ed.). New York: Appleton-Century-Crofts, p. 161.

◁ ——————————————————————————

progression, are derived from the multipotential hematopoietic stem cells **(CFU-S)** through the promonocyte **(PrMon),** the difference between monocytes and promonocytes being quite subtle. Monocytes may differentiate further into macrophages **(Mφ)** and later, by fusion, into multinucleate giant cells **(GC).** There is a stem cell *CFU-GM,* derived from the multipotential stem cell CFU-S, capable of differentiating either into the monocyte line or into the neutrophil line. It is not shown in this schema, but is discussed on p. 490.

Lymphocyte differentiation, presented in the lowermost progression, appears to depend on a lymphoid cell, a *lymphoblast* **(Lyb),** derived from the multipotential stem cell. The lymphoblast differentiates into a *T lymphoblast* **(Lyb-T),** which produces *T lymphocytes* **(Ly-T)** and *B lymphocytes* **(Ly-B).** When appropriately stimulated, as by antigen, T and B lymphocytes become larger and develop nucleoli, polyribosomes, and other organelles associated with protein synthesis and mitosis. These altered T and B lymphocytes are said to have undergone *"blast" formation* **(Lyb'-T** and **Lyb'-B).** They can go on to produce *plasma cells* **(PC)** and more **(Ly'-B)**-memory cells, in the case of B lymphocytes, and more **(Ly'-T)**-memory cells, in the case of T lymphocytes. The differentiation of CFUS into the lymphocyte lines is not evident (except in the case of plasma cells) in electron micrographs or in Romanovsky-stained material. Recognition of T and B cells depends on the visualization of distinctive cell-surface receptors by fluorescence microscopy or other means.

Basophilic Leukocytes

Dvorak, A. M. 1978. Biology and morphology of basophilic leukocytes. In Immediate Hypersensitivity, Modern Concepts and Development, Immunology Series, vol. 7, Bach, M. K. (ed.). New York: Marcel Dekker, Inc., p. 369.

Dvorak, A. M., Galli, S. J., Morgan, E., Galli, A. S., Hammond, M. E., and Dvorak, H. F. 1981. Anaphylactic degranulation of guinea pig basophilic leukocytes. I. Fusion of granule membranes and cytoplasmic vesicles: Formation and resolution of degranulation sacs. Lab. Invest. 44:174.

Terry, R. W., Bainton, D. F., and Farquhar, M. G. 1969. Formation and structure of specific granules in basophilic leukocytes of the guinea pig. Lab. Invest. 21:65.

Eosinophilic Leukocytes

Archer, G. T. 1963. Motion picture studies on degranulation of horse eosinophils during phagocytosis. J. Exp. Med. 118:276.

Beeson, P. B., and Bass, D. A. 1977. The eosinophil. Philadelphia: W. B. Saunders, Inc.

Erythrocytes

Brookoff, D., and Weiss, L. 1982. Adipocyte development and the loss of erythropoietic capacity in the bone marrow of mice after sustained hypertransfusion. Blood 60: December.

Harrison, P. R. 1976. Analysis of erythropoiesis at the molecular level. Review article. Nature (London) 262:353.

Howell, W. H. 1890. The life history of the formed elements of the blood: Especially the red corpuscles. J. Morphol. 4:57.

Johnson, G. R., and Metcalf, D. 1977c. Pure and mixed erythroid colony formation in vitro: Stimulation by spleen conditioned medium with no detectable erythropoietin. Proc. Natl. Acad. Sci. U.S.A. 74:3,879.

Rifkind, R. A., and Marks, P. A. 1975. The regulation of erythropoiesis. Blood Cells 1:417.

Lymphocytes

(See References and Selected Bibliography, Chapter 14 and Chapter 15)

Megakaryocytes and Platelets

Evatt, B. L., Levine, R. F., and Williams, N. T. 1981. Megakaryocyte Biology and Precursors: in vitro Cloning and Cellular Properties. New York: Elsevier-North Holland.

Metcalf, D., MacDonald, H. R., Odartchenki, N., and Sordat, B. 1975. Growth of mouse megakaryocyte colonies in vitro. Proc. Natl. Acad. Sci. U.S.A. 72:1744.

Paulus, J. M., Bury, J., and Grosent, J. C. 1979. Control of platelet territory development in megakaryocytes.

Penington, D. G. 1979. The cellular biology of megakaryocytes. Blood Cells 5:5.

Shattil, S. J., and Bennet, J. S. 1981. Platelets and their membranes in hemostasis: Physiology and pathophysiology. Ann. Intern. Med. 94:108.

Weissman, G., and Rite, G. A. 1972. Molecular basis of gouty inflammation: Interaction of monosodium urate crystals with lysosomes and liposomes. Nature (New Biol.) 240:167.

White, J. G., and Clawson, C. C. 1980. Overview article: Biostructure of blood platelets. Ultrastruct. Pathol. 1:533.

Williams, N., McDonald, T. P., and Trabellino, E. M. 1979. Maturation and regulation of megakaryocytopoiesis. Blood Cells 5:43.

Wright, J. H. 1910. The histogenesis of blood platelets. J. Morphol. 21:263.

Monocytes and Macrophages

(See References and Selected Bibliography, Chap. 4)

Neutrophilic Leukocytes

Bainton, D. F. Ullyot, J. L., and Farquhar, M. G. 1971. The development of neutrophilic polymorphonuclear leukocytes in human bone marrow. Origin and content of azurophil and specific granules. J. Exp. Med. 134:907.

Cohn, Z. A., and Morse, S. I. 1960. Functional and metabolic properties of polymorphonuclear leukocytes. I. Observations on the requirements and consequences of particle ingestion. J. Exp. Med. 111:667.

Craddock, C. G., Jr., Perry, S., Ventzke, L. E., and Lawrence, J. S. 1960. Evaluation of marrow granulocytic reserves in normal and disease states. Blood 15:840.

Hirsch, J. G., and Cohn, Z. A. 1960. Degranulation of polymorphonuclear leukocytes following phagocytosis of microorganisms. J. Exp. Med. 118:1005.

Johnson, G. R., and Metcalf, D. 1978. Characterization of mouse fetal liver granulocyte-macrophage colony-forming cells (GM-CFC) using velocity sedimentation. Exp. Hematol (Copenhagen). 6:246.

Johnson, G. R., and Metcalf, D. 1978. Sources and nature of granulocyte-macrophage colony stimulating factor in fetal mice. Exp. Hematol. (Copenhagen) 6:327.

Lisiewicz, J. 1980. Human Neutrophils. Bowe, Md.: The Charles Press Publishers.

Murphy, P. 1976. The Neutrophil. New York: Plenum.

Ramsey, W. A. 1972. Locomotion of human polymorphonuclear leukocytes. Exp. Cell Res. 72:489.

Spitznagel, J. K., Dalldorf, F. G., and Leffell, M. S. 1974. Characterization of azurophil and specific granules purified from human polymorphonuclear leukocytes. Lab. Invest. 30:774.

Weissman, G., and Rite, G. A. 1972. Molecular basis of gouty inflammation: Interaction of monosodium urate crystals with lysosomes and liposomes. Nature (New Biol.) 240:167.

Stem Cells

Abramson, S., Miller, R. G., and Phillips, R. A. 1977. Identification of pluripotent and restricted stem cells of the myeloid and lymphoid systems. J. Exp. Med. 145:1567.

van Bekkum, D. W., van Noord, M. J., Maat, B., and Dicke, K. A. 1971. Attempts at identification of hematopoietic stem cell in mouse. Blood 38:547.

Dexter, T. M., Allen, T. D., Lajtha, L. G., Krizsa, F., Testa, N. G., and Moore, M. A. S. 1978. In vitro analysis of self-renewal and commitment of hematopoietic stem cells. In Differentiation of normal and Neoplastic Hematopoietic Cells, Clarkson, B., Marks, P. A., Till, J. E., (eds.). Cold Spring Harbor Laboratory, New York: Vol A, p. 63.

Dicke, K. A., van Noord, M. J., and van Bekkum, D. W. 1973. Attempts at morphological identification of the hematopoietic stem cell in rodents and primates. Exp. Hemat. 1:36.

Donahue, D. M., Gabrio, B. W., and Finch, C. A. 1958. Quantitative measurements of hematopoietic cells of the marrow. J. Clin. Invest. 37:1,564.

Fowler, J. H., Wu, A. M., Till, J. E., McCulloch, E. A., and Siminovitch, L. 1967. The cellular composition of hematopoietic spleen colonies J. Cell Physiol. 69:65.

Johnson, G. R., and Moore, M. A. S. 1975. Role of stem cell migration in initiation of mouse foetal liver haemopoiesis. Nature (London) 258:726.

Moore, M. A. S., and Johnson, G. R. 1976. Stem cells during embryonic development and growth. In Cairnie, A. B., Lala, P. K., and Osmond, D. G. (eds.). Stem Cells of Renewing Cell Populations. New York: Academic Press, Inc., p. 323.

Moore, M. A. S., and Metcalf, D. 1970. Ontogeny of the haemopoietic system: Yolk sac origin of in vivo and in vitro colony forming cells in the developing mouse embryo. Br. J. Haematol. 18:279.

Siminovitch, L., McCulloch, E. A., and Till, J. E. 1963. The distribution of colony-forming cells among spleen colonies. J. Cell Comp. Physiol. 62:327.

Wu, A. M., Till, J. E., Siminovitch, L., and McCulloch, E. A. 1967. A cytological study of the capacity for differentiation of normal hematopoietic colony-forming cells. J. Cell Physiol. 69:177.

Wu, A. M., Till, J. E., Siminovitch, L., and McCulloch, E. A. 1968. Cytological evidence for a relationship between normal hematopoietic colony-forming cells and cells of the lymphoid system. J. Exp. Med. 127:455.

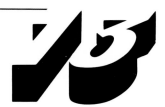

Bone Marrow

Leon Weiss

The bone marrow is a richly cellular connective tissue within the bones of the body, specialized to produce blood cells and deliver them to the circulation. It is the major hematopoietic tissue in human beings from the fifth month of fetal life through adulthood and accounts for about 5% of adult body weight. It attracts and holds hematopoietic stem cells in far greater number than any other tissue and provides diverse hematopoietic microenvironments for their maintenance and differentiation into each of the blood cell types. The differentiation of each of the blood cell types is initiated in the bone marrow. Erythrocytes, granulocytes, platelets, and monocytes develop almost completely in the marrow, with perhaps some terminal development occurring in the spleen before they are released to the general circulation. B lymphocytes undergo much of their development in marrow but mature in the spleen before entering the circulation. T lymphocyte development is initiated in marrow, occurs largely in the thymus, and is completed in the spleen.

Structure of Bone Marrow

Gross Characteristics

Bone marrow can be red, because of the presence of erythrocytes and their precursors, indicative of active hematopoiesis, or yellow, owing to fat and indicative of reduced hematopoiesis. Red and yellow marrow may be interconvertible, as demands for hematopoiesis change.

All marrow in newborn humans is red. Fat appears in long bones from the fifth to seventh years, and by the eighteenth year almost all limb marrow is yellow. Patches of red marrow persist only around the joints. Hematopoietic marrow in adults is virtually restricted to the skull, clavicles, vertebrae, ribs, sternebrae, and pelvis. Blood vessels and nerves reach marrow by piercing its bony shell. Particularly at the end of long bones, the internal surface of bone may be ridged with shelves and spicules of bone, the *trabeculae*, which protrude into the marrow cavity (Fig. 13–1).

Vascular Arrangements

There may be multiple small arterial twigs penetrating bone, or a major vessel, the *nutrient artery*, that enters marrow about midshaft in long bone and sends branches, *central longitudinal arteries*, that run in the central longitudinal axis of the marrow to the diaphyses. Slender branches of these arteries run radially through marrow toward the encasing bone and connect with venous vessels throughout the marrow cavity. Small arterial vessels actually enter the bone where they may become part of osteones or curve back toward the marrow and open into venous vessels.

The *venous* or *vascular sinuses* of marrow, the first vessels in the venous system, are thin-walled vessels 50 to 75 μm in diameter that anastomose richly. In long bones they run radially and empty into the central longitudinal vein, which runs in company with the corresponding artery (Figs. 13–2 to 13–4).

The circulation in marrow, in contrast to the spleen, is "closed" in that arteries connect directly to veins. Such direct connections have been demonstrated by vital microscopy and scanning electron microscopy (Fig. 13–5) and by the absence of blood from hematopoietic perivascular tissue.

The prominent system of venous sinuses and veins together with the system of arterial vessels constitutes the *vascular compartment* of the marrow. The remainder of the marrow lies between these vessels as irregular and anastomosing cords, the *hematopoietic cords*, and constitutes the *hematopoietic compartments* (Figs. 13–2 to 13–6). Hematopoiesis is most active in the periphery of the marrow near bone. Some fat always occurs in the center of the marrow in the hematopoietic compartment around the great vessels. In yellow marrow, the hematopoietic compartment is predominantly fatty.

Marrow lacks lymphatic vessels. The nerves in marrow are associated with the vasculature and appear to be vasomotor. The internal surface of the bone enclosing the marrow is lined with endosteum, composed of osteoblasts, osteoclasts and other bone lining cells (Chap. 6).

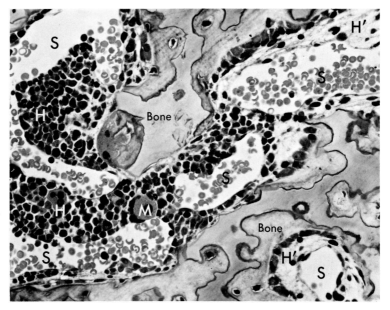

13–1 Bone marrow from central femur of human fetus, 200 mm crown rump length (22 weeks gestational age). The marrow tissue occurs in the spaces within bone. In the adult the bone will be removed from much of the center of the shaft of the femur, remaining only to form a cortical shell. The marrow will therefore become a solid cylindrical plug of tissue. The marrow contains large, thin-walled vascular sinuses **(S)** containing blood. Outside the sinuses lie the hematopoietic compartments. Some of them **(H)** are filled with hematopoietic cells. Note the large megakaryocyte **(M)** characteristically set on the outside wall of the sinus (see text). In some sites, the hematopoietic compartments have not yet filled with hematopoietic cells but contain fibrous connective tissue **(H')**. × 1,000. (From L-T. Chen and L. Weiss.)

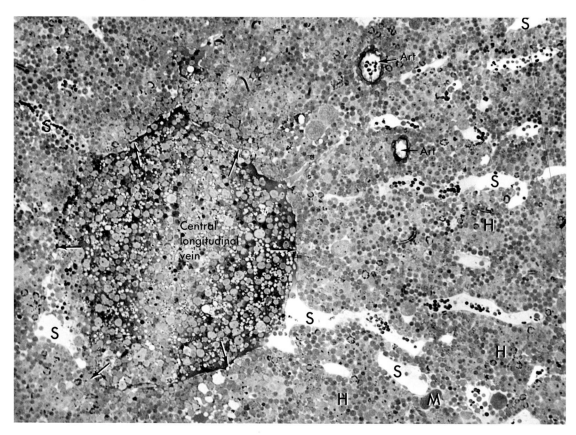

13–2 Rat bone marrow. This is a cross section of the marrow showing the relationships of major structural elements. The central longitudinal vein and branches of the nutrient artery **(Art)** are cut in cross section. The lumen of the vein is filled with cells: its wall is indicated by **arrows.** The sinuses **(S)** constitute a thin-walled radial system of venous vessels running into the vein. They are cut in longitudinal section. They are separated by hematopoietic compartments **(H)** containing the developing blood cells packed together. Megakaryocytes **(M)** lie characteristically against the outside wall of a sinus. × 750. (From Weiss, L. 1965. J. Morphol. 117:481.)

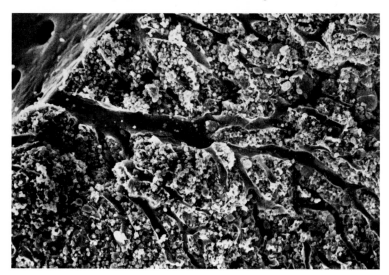

13–3 Rat bone marrow. This is a scanning electron micrograph of the cut surface showing a system of vascular sinuses originating at the periphery of the marrow (right side of field) and draining into a large vein (left upper corner). The large vein has several apertures in its wall, representing the entry of tributary venous sinuses. Hematopoietic tissue lies between the vascular sinuses. × 800. (From Weiss, L. 1976. Anat. Rec. 186:161.)

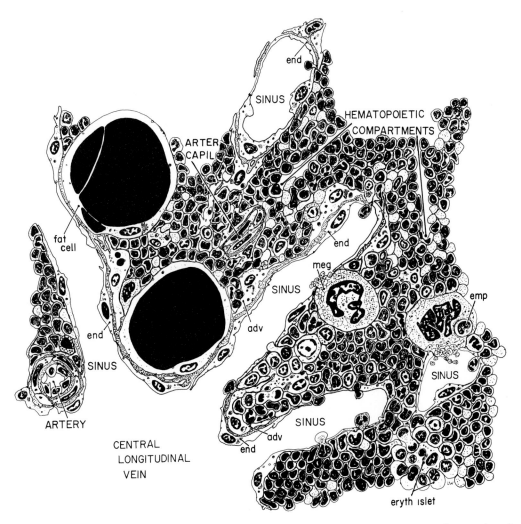

13–4 Bone marrow, schematic view of cross section near central longitudinal vein. Several sinuses drain into the central longitudinal vein. The sinuses are cut along their long axis, the vein, in cross section. A portion of the nutrient artery is present, as is an arterial capillary. Hematopoietic cells lie between the sinuses, constituting the hematopoietic compartment. Where hematopoiesis is relatively quiet, the wall of the sinus and of the central longitudinal vein is trilaminar consisting of endothelium **(end),** a basement membrane, and adventitial cell **(adv).** The adventitial cell may become voluminous, encroaching upon the hematopoietic space and thereby displacing hematopoietic cells. The increased volume of the adventitial cell may be due to a gelatinous change wherein its cytoplasm becomes rarefied, presumably because of hydration. If this change is widespread, the marrow may become grossly white and gelatinous. A second and more common basis for the large bulk of adventitial cells is fatty change, where they become fat cells. Contrariwise, when hematopoiesis is active the hematopoietic compartment is large and packed with myelocytes, erythroblasts, and megakaryocytes. The sinus wall becomes thin, reduced to an endothelial layer alone as the adventitial cells are displaced or lifted from the wall by infiltrating hematopoietic cells. Apertures appear in the endothelium, moreover, as maturing hematopoietic cells cross the sinus wall and enter the sinus lumen. Megakaryocytes **(meg)** characteristically lie against the outside of the sinus wall, discharging platelets into the lumen through an aperture. Occasionally the cytoplasm of megakaryocytes is entered by other cell types, which remain visible and later leave the megakaryocyte. The phenomenon is known as emperipolesis **(emp).** Erythroblasts tend to be present in clusters near the sinus wall. Erythroblastic islets (see text) may be present. Granulocytes usually develop near the center of the hematopoietic space. Lymphocytes occur throughout the marrow. Macrophages are common, and mast cells, plasma cells, and other connective tissue cells are also present.

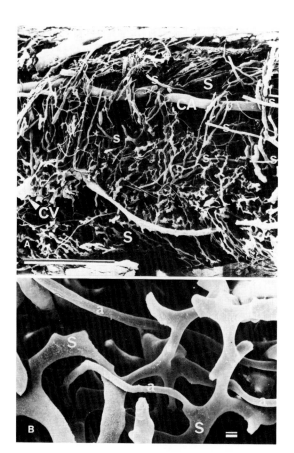

13–5 **A.** A scanning electron micrograph of the vascular cast of longitudinally cut rat's femur. Numerous fine terminal arterioles are seen arising from side branches **(s)** of the central artery **(CA). CV,** cut edge of the central vein; **S,** marrow sinusoid. Bar = 1 mm. **B.** A closer view of the vascular cast of the rat's bone marrow. Two terminal arterioles **(a)** are seen connecting with the sinusoids **(S).** Bar = 10 μm. (From the work of Osamu Ohtani.)

Vascular Sinuses

Blood cells are produced in the hematopoietic compartments and reach the circulation by crossing the wall of vascular sinuses. The sinus wall is therefore the barrier between hematopoietic tissue and the blood. In its fullest development the wall has three layers: endothelium, basement membrane, and adventitia (Figs. 13–4, and 13–6 to 13–9).

The endothelium is a thin, simple layer of flat cells connected to one another by circumferential zonulae adherens, probably associated with gap junctions. Endothelial cells contain many small vesicles, microfilaments, microtubules,

some ribosomes, small Golgi complexes, lysosomes, and heterolysosomes. The basement membrane is variably seen both because it may be absent physiologically, and because, when present, it is difficult to preserve by most electron-microscopic methods. Adventitial cells normally cover most of the outside surface of the endothelium. In the femoral marrow of the rat, more than 60% is covered. Adventitial cells vary in appearance but contain most of the organelles present in endothelium. These cells lie on the outside surface of the vascular sinuses as the most peripheral of the vascular layers and branch out into the surrounding hematopoietic cords. By their branching they form a meshwork, which supports the hematopoietic cells of the cords. The adventitial cells are therefore related to the reticular meshworks in the splenic cords and in lymph nodes, except that reticular fibers in marrow are much slighter and may be absent. Hence, the adventitial cells are a type of reticular cell and are termed *adventitial reticular cells*.

The reticular meshwork of the hematopoietic cords holds the developing blood cells. Reticular cells may play a further role in sorting hematopoietic cells into characteristic locations. They may well contribute to the hematopoietic microenvironments of marrow and thereby influence hematopoietic differentiation.

Adventitial reticular cells may become swollen, voluminous, and "empty" in appearance, probably because of marked water uptake. If this change occurs on a large scale, the marrow may become grossly white and gelatinous. Adventitial reticular cells, moreover, may become fatty; when this occurs extensively, the marrow becomes yellow (Figs. 13–4 and 13–9). These gelatinous or fatty cells protrude deeply into the perivascular hematopoietic cord and decrease the space available for hematopoiesis. Gelatinous or fatty marrows, therefore, are reduced in hematopoietic activity. As indicated above, the marrow is normally yellow in certain locations, as in the appendicular skeleton; but after exposure to certain toxins, normally hematopoietic red marrow may become fatty, resulting in reduced marrow hematopoietic capacity and anemia *(aplastic anemia)*. In contrast, when hematopoietic volume must increase, as it does in response to severe blood loss and in certain diseases (such as leukemia or infection), it displaces normally fatty marrow. The fatty adventitial cells lose their fat, thereby decreasing in volume and providing additional space for hematopoiesis. Gelat-

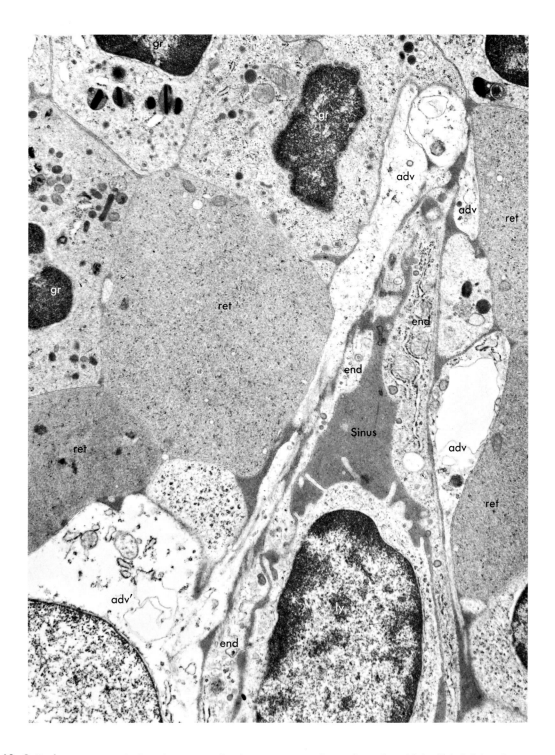

13–6 Rat bone marrow. A sinus is present, closely surrounded by hematopoietic cells. The lumen of the sinus contains a lymphocyte **(ly).** Its wall consists of endothelial **(end)** and adventitial **(adv)** layers. At the lower left corner of the field, the cytoplasm of an adventitial cell **(adv′)** is voluminous and extends into the surrounding hematopoietic space. Reticulocytes **(ret)** and granulocytes **(gr)** surround the sinus. × 15,200. (From Weiss, L. 1970. Blood 36:189.)

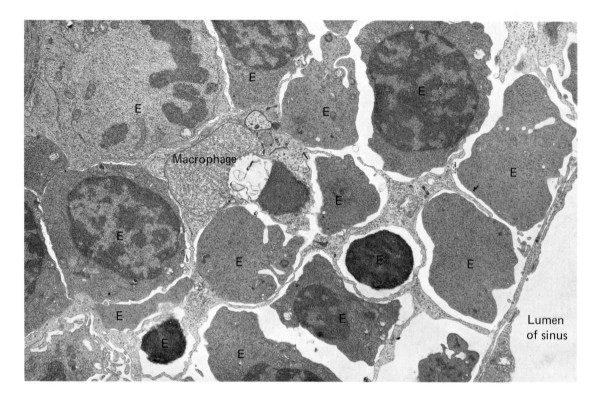

13–7 Rat bone marrow, erythroblastic islet. A macrophage lies amid a cluster of red cells **(E)**. It sends out a system of slender branching cell processes that enclose the surrounding red cells and reach to the wall of a vascular sinus on the upper right. (This tissue was perfused and the cells, as a result, are separated from one another, thereby revealing the extensive branching of the macrophage clearly.) × 7,300. (From Weiss, L. 1976. Anat. Rec. 186:161.)

inous and fatty transformations of adventitial reticular cells constitute mechanisms to change the volume of hematopoietic space in an organ which, because its "capsule" is bone, does not readily change and which, therefore must have a rather constant total volume.[1]

Fat cells do more than control hematopoietic space. They are active in the metabolism of steroid hormones, aromatizing testosterone to estrogens, as shown by Frisch. It also appears from Dexter's studies of bone marrow in tissue culture that fat cells induce granulocyte differentiation.

---

[1]In certain pathological states where hematopoiesis is abnormally intense for long periods, the bone in trabeculae and the cortex may thin considerably, even breaking as a result of minor trauma (pathological fracture).

The Hematopoietic Compartment

The hematopoietic tissue in marrow lies between vascular sinuses and consists of hematopoietic cells, mast cells, and related cell types of connective tissue held in a reticular meshwork formed by branches of reticular cells. The relative numbers of nucleated marrow hematopoietic cells are given in Table 13–1.

There is a pattern to the arrangement of hematopoietic cells in the hematopoietic compartments. Megakaryocytes lie close against the adventitial surface of vascular sinuses (Figs. 13–1, 13–2, and 13–4). They lie over apertures in the vascular wall and discharge platelets directly into the lumen. By lying over such an aperture, the megakaryocyte efficiently delivers platelets into the vascular lumen and, by its large size, both resists being swept into the circulation and prevents vascular leakage.

Erythrocytes are produced near sinuses. As they mature to the point where nuclear polarization is marked (Fig. 12–7) the cytoplasmic pole is typically directed toward a vascular sinus. Nuclear and cytoplasmic poles separate, and the cytoplasmic portion, now a freshly produced reticulocyte, remains near the wall. It becomes part of the reticulocyte reserve of the mar-

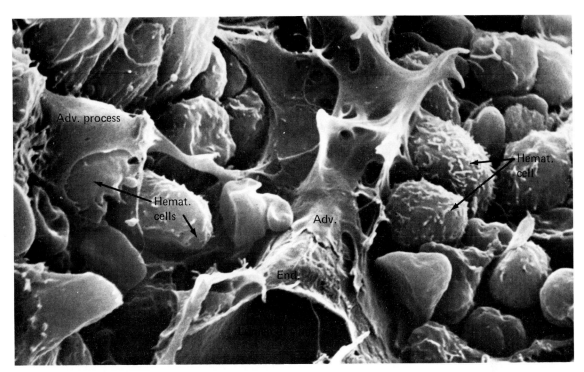

13–8 Rat bone marrow, scanning electron micrograph. A vascular sinus opens at the lower margin. The outside surface of its endothelium **(End)** is clothed by a reticular cell in adventitial position **(Adv)** in the vascular wall. The adventitial cell branches into the surrounding hematopoietic tissue. On the left a branch **(Adv process)** partially envelops a hematopoietic cell **(Hemat cell).** On the right, two hematopoietic cells bearing microvilli press against the outside surface of the vessel. Cells appear to develop microvilli preparatory to passing across the vascular wall into the lumen. × 4,000. (From Weiss, L. 1976. Anat. Rec. 186:161.)

13–9 Rat bone marrow, scanning electron micrograph. A sinus lies at the right, with the luminal surface of its endothelium **(End surface)** and the torn edge of its endothelium **(End edge)** on view. The adventitial reticular cells have become fatty **(Fat cell)** and extend into the hematopoietic space, occupying space that would otherwise be available for hematopoiesis. × 4,050. (From Weiss, L. 1976. Anat. Rec. 186:161.)

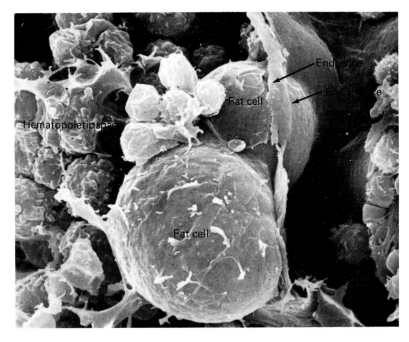

Table 13–1 Relative Number of Nucleated Cells in Normal Bone Marrow

	Range	Average
Myeloblasts	0.3–5.0	2.0
Promyelocytes	1.0–8.0	5.0
Myelocytes		
Neutrophilic	5.0–19.0	12.0
Eosinophilic	0.5–3.0	1.5
Basophilic	0.0–0.5	0.3
Metamyelocytes ("juvenile" forms)	13.0–32.0	22.0
Polymorphonuclear neutrophils	7.0–30.0	20.0
Polymorphonuclear eosinophils	0.5–4.0	2.0
Polymorphonuclear basophils	0.0–0.7	0.2
Lymphocytes	3.0–17.0	10.0
Plasma cells	0.0–2.0	0.4
Monocytes	0.5–5.0	2.0
Reticular cells	0.1–2.0	0.2
Megakaryocytes	0.03–3.0	0.4
Pronormoblasts	1.0–8.0	4.0
Erythroblasts (basophilic, polychromatophilic, and acidophilic)	7.0–32.0	18.0

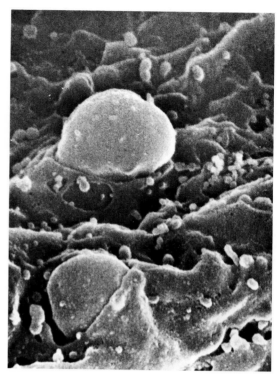

13–10 Rat bone marrow, scanning electron micrograph. This is a view of a vascular sinus on its luminal surface. Two cells are passing through the endothelium, probably entering the lumen of the sinus and the circulation. The upper cell is constricted as it squeezes through the endothelium. The lower one has a cowl of endothelium around it as it appears to emerge. × 3,000. (From Weiss, L., and Chen, L.-T. 1975. Blood cells, 1:617.)

row; after a variable time, an aperture in the wall is formed, and the reticulocyte squeezes through into the lumen of the sinus. Alternatively, a reticulocyte can be released to the circulation as it is being produced. The nuclear pole is phagocytized (Chap. 12). Macrophages are regularly associated with developing erythroblasts, phagocytizing nuclear poles, secreting factors that regulate erythropoiesis, and, perhaps, facilitating the delivery of reticulocytes to the circulation. Macrophages may lie among erythroblasts in no apparent arrangement, but often a macrophage lies in the center of an *erythroblastic islet,* its cytoplasm extending out and enclosing surrounding erythroblasts (Fig. 13–7). There may be one or more circlets or tiers of erythroblasts in an islet. The outer tiers consist of more mature cells than do the inner ones. Other cell types are associated with erythropoiesis, particularly when it is heightened as, for example, in response to severe blood loss. Then characteristic branched dense stromal cells and lymphocytes may be seen in company with macrophages and erythroblasts.

Granulocytes are typically produced in nests or as dispersed sheets of cells, somewhat away from the vascular sinus. On maturation, at the metamyelocyte stage, they become motile and join the reserve of marrow granulocytes, ready to move toward the vascular sinus and exit across

the wall of the sinus into the circulation (Figs. 13–10 and 13–11). As granulocyte precursors mature, they are regularly associated with other cell types. This is seen clearly during heightened granulocytopoiesis as, for example, in the intensified eosinophilopoiesis that occurs after infection with the nematode worm *Ascaris suum.* Then branched stromal cells, macrophages, and lymphocytes similar to those attending heightened erythropoiesis are present in proximity to the eosinophils (Fig. 13–12).

Delivery of Blood Cells to the Circulation

Maturing blood cells move from the hematopoietic compartment into the circulation through apertures in the walls of vascular sinuses. As

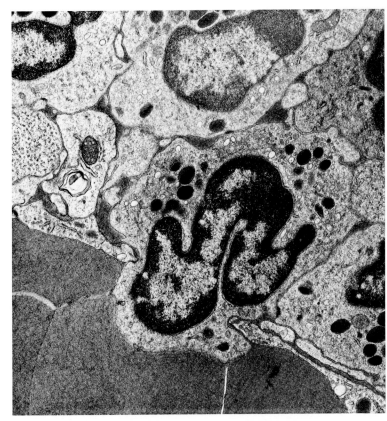

13-11 Mouse bone marrow. An eosinophil is crossing the wall of a vascular sinus, passing from the hematopoietic compartment above into the blood, below. × 9,500. (From N. Sakai and L. Weiss.)

blood cells mature they move to the adventitial surface of the vascular sinus. Adventitial cells move away from the wall, and the basement membrane depolymerizes, leaving the endothelium as the only barrier to the lumen of the sinus. The maturing blood cells press against the basal surface of the endothelium and apertures appear in the endothelial cells near (but not at) endothelial cell junctions. The blood cells then squeeze through into the lumen of the sinus. Apertures normally develop only in relationship to cell passage; they are either occupied by a cell in transit or absent. The integrity of the endothelial barrier between blood and hematopoietic compartments is thereby maintained (Figs. 13–4, 13–10, and 13–11).

Hematopoietic Microenvironment

Several lines of evidence suggest that hematopoietic organs provide a distinctive microenvironment that can influence the differentiation of blood cells. When an animal whose hematopoietic tissues have been destroyed by irradia-

tion is given a suspension of multipotential hematopoietic stem cells (CFU-S), the stem cells "home" to the hematopoietic tissues and, by proliferating and differentiating there, restore hematopoietic activity. The CFU-Ss going to the spleen differentiate mostly into erythroblasts, whereas those going to bone marrow differentiate into granulocytes and macrophages and, to a lesser extent, erythroblasts. Within the spleen and bone marrow, moreover, there are separate zones that favor erythroid, lymphocytic, or granulocytic differentiation. A pair of mouse congenital anemias further supports the concept of the hematopoietic microenvironment. The Wv/Wv strain of mouse has a mild anemia due to a deficiency in CFU-Ss; when stem cells are provided the anemia is cured. However, in the clinically similar anemia of the Sl/Sl^d mouse there are normal numbers of CFU-Ss, as shown by spleen colony assay, and the anemia cannot be cured by administering hematopoietic cells. The deficiency in this animal is considered to be due to a defect in the stroma, vasculature, or associated cells—in short, to the microenvironment.

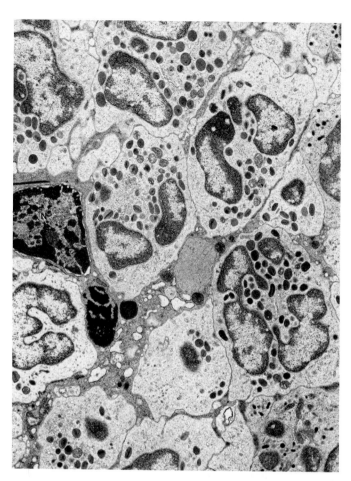

13–12 Mouse bone marrow stimulated to heightened eosinophilopoiesis. Many eosinophils in various stages of differentiation lie in the field. A large, branched stromal cell extends among them, its nucleus (N). A similar stromal cell may be found among developing blood cells during heightened hematopoiesis affecting any blood cell type. (From Weiss, L., and Sakai, N. 1981. Microenvironments in hematopoietic and lymphoid differentiation, London: Pitman.)

Pathology

Hematopoietic activity of bone marrow may increase (hyperplasia) or decrease (hypoplasia or aplasia). Such change may affect every blood cell type or selected types. Increased hematopoietic activity may be due to an increase of essentially normal cells (such as in increased production of red cells after hemorrhage) or to abnormal cells (such as in the leukemias). In the leukemias, abnormal leukocytes are produced and may crowd the normal cells out. Leukemias occur in the different white blood cell types, as monocytic leukemia, lymphocytic leukemia, and so forth. A related malignancy of bone marrow is *multiple myeloma*. Here the marrow is crowded with myeloma cells that represent abnormal plasma cells. The myeloma cells in any given case constitute a clone that produces an abnormal incomplete antibody molecule. Knowledge of the amino acid sequence of such molecules has been valuable for elucidating normal antibody structure.

In *polycythemia vera* there is hypertrophy of the erythroblastic mass but the number of leukocytes and megakaryocytes may also be increased. Erythropoiesis may be so intense in certain anemias (as in the thalassemias) that the internal surface of the bone is eroded and trabeculae become reduced in size and number as the marrow cavity expands. Despite this considerable increase in erythropoiesis, the number of erythrocytes in the circulation is usually quite low because the erythrocytes in these conditions are markedly defective cells with considerably shortened life spans. There are many animal models of hematological disease. A congenital hemolytic anemia in the deer mouse appears similar to a congenital hemolytic anemia in children. Hemolytic anemias due to spectrin deficiencies have been shown in mice and in human beings.

In contrast, the bone marrow may become hypoplastic. Marrow may be reduced to a fatty state by starvation. Many chemicals are toxic to marrow. Lead and benzene may produce an aplastic anemia. Certain toxins may be used therapeutically, such as the nitrogen mustards, which suppress or destroy abnormal bone marrow like that in leukemia. Aplastic anemia may be genetically determined, and some animal models, such as the Wv/Wv and Sl/Sl^d strains discussed above, are providing insight into the mechanisms. In a rare human condition, the Diamond-Blackfan syndrome of congenital aplastic anemia, T_s lymphocytes may suppress erythropoiesis. Malignant tumors may metastasize to bone marrow and create aplastic marrows by suppressing or displacing normal hematopoietic tissue. In some instances, vascular sinuses may become widely dilated with blood, encroaching on hematopoietic tissue and, paradoxically, conferring a brilliant red color on a hematopoietically inactive tissue. Hormones and humoral substances in addition to those (such as erythropoietin) specifically directed toward hematopoietic tissues influence hematopoiesis. Estrogens inhibit erythropoiesis and testosterone stimulates it. Unchecked production of calcitonin may result in bony overgrowth and a decrease in the volume of the marrow cavity, leading to a reduced output of blood cells.

References and Selected Bibliography

General

Bloom, W., and Bartelmez, G. W., 1940. Hematopoiesis in young human embryos. Am. J. Anat. 67:21.

Bråanemark, P. I. 1959. Vital microscopy of bone marrow in rabbit. Scand. J. Clin. Lab. Invest. (Suppl. 38) 11:1.

Donahue, D. M., Gabrio, B. W., and Finch, C. A. 1958. Quantitative measurement of hematopoietic cells of the marrow. J. Clin. Invest. 37:1564.

Gilmour, J. R. 1941. Normal hematopoiesis in intrauterine and neonatal life. J. Pathol. Bact. 52:25.

Weiss, L. 1965. The structure of bone marrow. Functional interrelationships of vascular and hematopoietic compartments in experimental hemolytic anemia. J. Morphol. 117:481.

Weiss, L. 1972. The Cells and Tissues of the Immune System. Englewood Cliffs, N.J.: Prentice-Hall.

Weiss, L., and Chen, L. T. 1975. The organization of hematopoietic cords and vascular sinuses in bone marrow. Blood Cells 1:617.

Wickramasinghe, S. N. 1975. Human Bone Marrow. Oxford: Blackwell Scientific Publications, Ltd.

Hematopoiesis

Allen, T. D., and Dexter, T. M. 1976. Cellular interrelationships during in vitro granulopoiesis. Differentiation. 6:191.

Huggins, C., and Blocksom, B. H. 1936. Changes in outlying bone marrow accompanying a local increase of temperature with physiological limits. J. Exp. Med. 64:253.

Iscove, N. N. 1977. The role of erythropoietin in regulation of population size and cell cycling of early and late erythroid precursors in mouse bone marrow. Cell Tissue Kinet. 10:323.

Lichtman, M. A. 1979. Cellular deformability during maturation of the myeloblast. Possible role in marrow egress. N. Engl. J. Med. 283:943.

Sakai, N., Johnstone, C., and Weiss, L. 1981. Bone marrow cells associated with heightened eosinophilopoiesis: An electron microscope study of murine bone marrow stimulated by Ascaris suum. Am. J. Anat. 161:11.

Trentin, J. J. 1970. Influence of hemopoietic organ stroma (hematopoietic inductive microenvironments) on stem cell differentiation. In Regulation of Hematopoiesis, vol. I: Red Cell Production, Gordon, A. S. (ed.). New York: Appleton-Crofts, p. 161.

Stroma

LaPushin, R. W., and Trentin, J. J., 1977. Identification of distinctive stromal elements in erythroid and neutrophil granuloid spleen colonies: Light and electron microscopic study. Exp. Hemat. 5:505.

McCuskey, R. S., and Meinke, H. A., 1973. Studies of the hematopoietic microenvironment. III. Differences in the splenic microvascular system and stroma between Sl/Sl^d and W/W^v mice. Am. J. Anat. 137:187.

Tavassoli, M. 1976. Marrow adipose cells-histochemical identification of labile and stable components. Arch. Pathol. Lab. Med. 100:16.

Weiss, L. 1976. The hematopoietic microenvironment of the bone marrow:An Ultrastructural study of the stroma in rats. Anat. Rec. 186:161.

Vasculature

Campbell, F. 1972. Ultrastructural studies of transmural migration of blood cells in the bone marrow of rats, mice and guinea pigs. Am. J. Anat. 135:521.

Doan, C. A. 1922. The capillaries of the bone marrow of the adult pigeon. Bull. Johns Hopkins Hosp. 33:222.

Fleidner, T. M. 1956. Research on the architecture of the vascular bed of the bone marrow of rats. Z. Zellforsch. Mikrosk. Anat. 45:328.

Lichtman, M. A., Chamberlain, J. K., and Santillo, P. A. 1978. Factors thought to contribute to the regulation of the egress of cells from marrow. In The Year in Hematology, Gordon, A. S., Silber, R. and Lobue, J. (eds.). New York: Plenum, p. 243.

Zamboni, L., and Pease, D. C. 1961. The vascular bed of red bone marrow. J. Ultrastruct. Res. 5:65.

Pathology

Hoshi, H., and Weiss, L. 1978. Rabbit bone marrow after administration of saponin. Lab. Invest. 38:67.

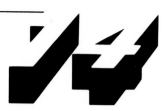

The Thymus

Leon Weiss

The human thymus is a lymphoepithelial organ derived both from the epithelium of the third branchial pouch and from lymphoid stem cells that enter from the blood. It is pyramidal, rests on the pericardium in the superior mediastinum, and achieves its greatest absolute weight, approximately 40 g, at puberty. It is bilaterally symmetrical, consisting of halves that meet in the midline except at the apex, where it extends into the neck and diverges around the trachea.

The thymus produces the T lymphocytes of the body from stem cells that migrate to it via the circulation from the bone marrow. The stem cells enter the thymus, proliferate, and mature there, presumably under the influence of the epithelial cells. The thymus also appears to monitor T-cell production, destroying those T cells capable of attacking self, that is, the body's own tissues, in contrast to foreign substances, such as bacteria or grafts or genetically different tissues. T cells are released by the thymus to complete their maturation in the spleen or lymph nodes. They then circulate and recirculate through the body, accumulating in spleen, lymph nodes, and other lymphatic tissues. Because the thymus does not itself directly participate to a significant degree in immune reactions, but rather releases cells to other tissues that do, it is, like bone marrow, classified as a *central immune organ*.

The thymus develops early compared with other lymphatic organs. It is well developed before birth, and before puberty it is round and fleshy. After puberty the thymus begins a remarkable *involution* or atrophy, its parenchyma

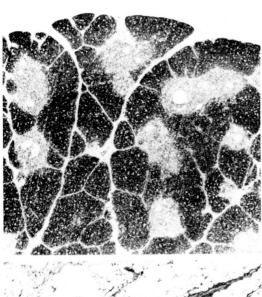

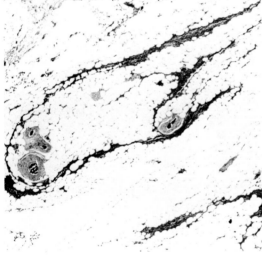

14–1 Human thymus before and after involution. The tissue in the **upper** micrograph is from an infant 3 mos. old; the **lower**, from a 72-year-old person. Note the lobular pattern in the upper micrograph. The medulla is a branching structure. The cortex surrounds the lobular projections of the medulla. A thin fibrous capsule is present. Involutional changes are evident in the lower micrograph. The cortex is markedly diminished, and the organ is fatty. The blood vessels display thickened sclerotic walls (see Fig. 14–12). × 25. (From the work of Robert Rouse.)

being gradually replaced by fatty and fibrous tissue (Fig. 14–1). This *age involution* may be greatly accelerated by certain types of stress; it is then called *accidental involution*. (See section on Involution, page 521.)

Structure of the Thymus

The thymus is divided into lobes and lobules by septae that extend into the organ from the surrounding connective tissue capsule. The lobules, 0.5 to 2.0 mm in length, are roughly rectangular in outline. Each lobule is divided into a peripheral zone relatively rich in lymphocytes, called the *cortex*, and a central zone relatively rich in epithelial cells, called the *medulla* (Figs. 14–1 and 14–2).

Major Cell Types

Epithelial Cells. Epithelial cells assume several forms in the thymus. A major epithelial conformation is a meshwork or *cytoreticulum* made of richly branched cells attached to one another by desmosomes. In contrast to the reticulum of mesenchymal organs such as the spleen, this meshwork is made of epithelial cells alone, without reticular fibers, and the cells are called *epithelial-reticular cells*. The interstices of this cytoreticulum are tightly packed with lymphocytes, and the plasma membrane of each lymphocyte is closely surrounded by the plasma membrane of an epithelial cell (Fig. 14–3). Epithelial-reticular cells have tonofilaments and desmosomes indicative of their epithelial character, and membrane-bounded cytoplasmic inclusions suggesting a secretory capacity. Indeed epithelial cells produce *thymosin* and other humoral factors that control thymic function (see below). Although epithelial-reticular cells are best seen in the cortex, which contains 95% of the lymphocytes of the thymus, they are also present (less fully branched) in the medulla. Epithelial cell sacs that completely enclose clusters of 50 or more lymphocytes are reported in the cortex of the thymus. They are saclike structures that have been found after disruption of the thymus and are quite difficult to visualize in sectioned material. It is possible, however, that the sacs are artifacts caused by disruption.

Another major group of epithelial cells forms *thymic corpuscles*, or *Hassall's corpuscles*, structures unique to the medulla (Figs. 14–2, and 14–5 to 14–7). When well developed, these corpuscles consist of epithelial cells rather tightly wound upon one another in a concentric pattern. The central cells are prone to become swollen, calcified, and necrotic. They may undergo lysis, leaving a cystic structure. The corpuscle may become markedly keratinized, resembling the epi-

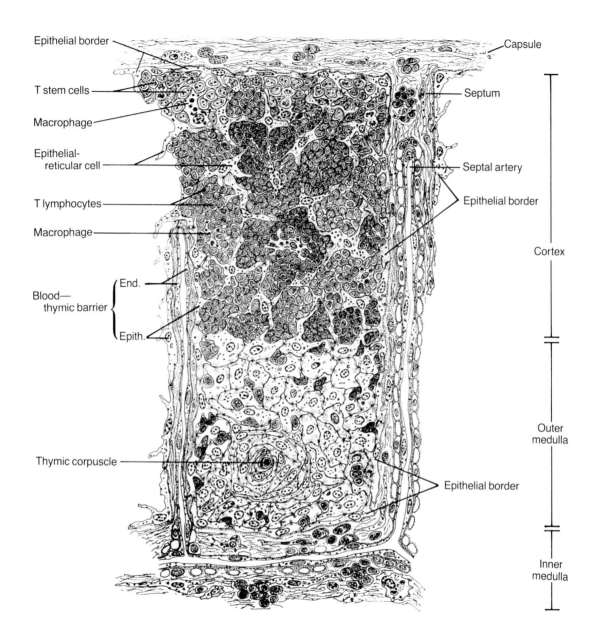

Epithelial border

T stem cells

Macrophage

Epithelial-
reticular cell

T lymphocytes

Macrophage

Blood—
thymic barrier { End.

Epith.

Thymic corpuscle

Capsule

Septum

Septal artery

Epithelial border

Cortex

Epithelial border

Outer
medulla

Inner
medulla

14–2 Schema of portion of thymus lobule. The cortex is heavily infiltrated with lymphocytes. As a result, the epithelial cells become stellate and remain attached to one another by desmosomes. The medulla is closer to a pure epithelium, although it, too, is commonly infiltrated by lymphocytes. A large thymic corpuscle, consisting of concentrically arranged epithelial cells, is shown. The capsule and trabeculae are rich in connective tissue fibers (mainly collagen) and contain blood vessels and variable numbers of plasma cells, granulocytes, and lymphocytes. A border of somewhat flattened epithelial cells surrounds the cortex and outer medulla.

dermis. Lymphocytes, eosinophils, and macrophages—usually degenerated—may lie within a thymic corpuscle. The peripheral epithelial cells within a corpuscle blend into the cytoreticulum. A thymic corpuscle may actually be present as a single cell, swollen, calcified, and degenerated, or it may be a huge multiform structure several hundred microns in one direction. Thymic corpuscles are well developed in human beings, dogs, and guinea pigs, and poorly developed in mice and rats. The number of thymic corpuscles in human beings reaches its maximum at about they surround blood vessels and make up a major component of the blood–thymic barrier (Figs. 14–8 to 14–12 and see below). They also lie along the perimeter of the gland, forming a slender epithelial border that encloses both the cortex and the medulla and thereby "seals off" the thymus from many outside influences (Fig. 14–2 and see below).

Lymphocytes. Before its involution, the thymus contains vast numbers of developing T lymphocytes. More than 95% of them lie in the cortex, dominating its appearance. Approximately 10% of thymic lymphocytes are large. These cells are concentrated in the outer cortex beneath

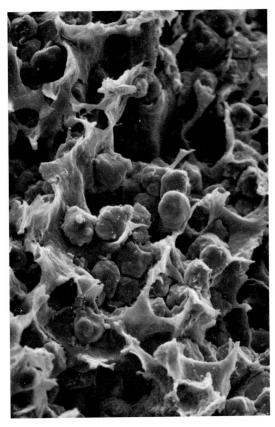

14–3 Rat thymus cortex, scanning electron micrograph. Many cortical lymphocytes have been washed away, revealing the broad branchings of the epithelial-reticular cells. Note that some of the lymphocytes remain, lying on the epithelial-reticular cells. × 5,700. (From the work of L.-T. Chen, B. W. Wetzel, and L. Weiss.)

14–4 Human thymus, infant. In this field a large epithelial cell **(Epith. cell)** lies among lymphocytes **(Ly)**. The surface of the epithelial cell reacts positively **(arrows)** in a cytochemical reaction labeling the Dr region of the major histocompatibility complex (the HLA complex in humans). The reaction depends on a monoclonal antibody reactive against the cell-surface antigens determined by the Dr region of the HLA complex. This antibody is linked to a horseradish peroxidase marker as discussed in Chap. 2. The HLA antigens on the surface of thymus cells are probably important in the cellular interactions underlying T-cell maturation and homing. See text for discussion. (From the work of Robert Rouse)

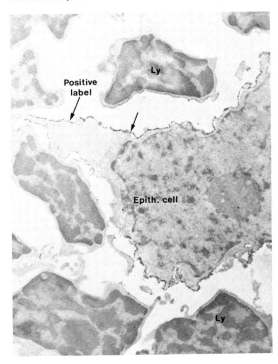

the time of puberty; from then on, they decrease in number, especially the smaller ones. With age, however, the remaining corpuscles become larger, and, as the thymus involutes, more prominent. The functions of thymic corpuscles are not known.

Epithelial cells in the thymus may occur as a simple cuboidal epithelium or a columnar ciliated mucus-producing epithelium lining the walls of cysts. Cysts are occasionally present in adult human thymus and may represent remnants of diverticuli of the fourth branchial pouches.

Epithelial cells in the thymus may also assume a barrier function. Somewhat flattened, and linked to one another by junctional complexes,

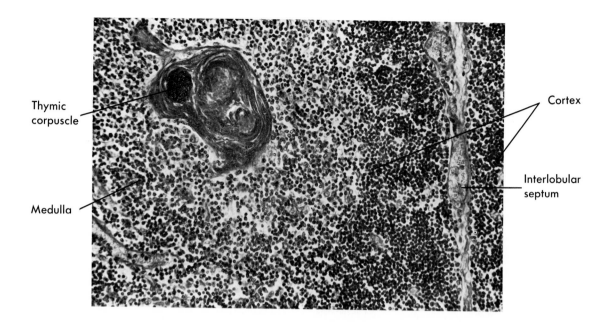

14–5 Thymus of a 20-year-old person. Lymphocytes are concentrated in the cortex. They are present in the medulla as well but are scattered loosely among epithelial-reticular cells. A large, multicentric thymic corpuscle is present in the medulla. The interlobular septum is slender and contains lymphatic vessels, blood vessels, and nerves. × 200. (Preparation from B. Castleman.)

the capsule and they actively proliferate. They represent stem cells recently arrived from bone marrow. The deeper part, and the bulk of the cortex, contains small thymic lymphocytes, about 85% of all thymic lymphocytes. They are maturing cells derived from the large subcapsular lymphocytes. As they mature they move deeper into the cortex, so that lymphocytes at the cortical–medullary junction and in the medulla are the most mature. Approximately 5% of thymic lymphocytes lie among the epithelial cells of the medulla. As thymic lymphocytes mature, they acquire distinctive markers on the cell surface and within the cytoplasm that are revealed by special staining. By standard light and electron-microscopic stains, developing T cells look like other lymphocytes. Small thymic lymphocytes, however, are somewhat smaller than small lymphocytes found elsewhere in the body. Degenerating lymphocytes are numerous but inconspicuous throughout the thymus. They may lie free or may be phagocytized by macrophages.

The kinetics of T-lymphocyte development can be followed by autoradiography after a single injection or pulse of tritiated thymidine. Lymphocytes in the outer cortex are labeled within 15 to 30 min. A shift of labeled cells then occurs, for in 12 to 24 h lymphocytes in the deep cortex and medulla become maximally labeled and the labeling of subcapsular lymphocytes is quite decreased. The total generation time of most thymic lymphocytes is about 9 h. The G_1 period is thought to be quite short. Thus the maturation of T lymphocytes, including their proliferation, differentiation, and migration from the subcapsular regions into the medulla, may occur within 24 h. Mature T lymphocytes leave the thymus by way of blood vessels and lymphatics.

Other Cells. Macrophages are invariably present within the thymus, lying among lymphocytes and epithelial cells of cortex and medulla. In addition to their evident phagocytic capacity, macrophages may secrete factors that stimulate T-cell mitosis or differentiation.

Antigen-presenting cells, similar to those present in white pulp of spleen and cortex of lymph nodes and related to the Langerhans cells of epidermis, are present in the thymic medulla. They bear Ia antigens on their surface and can contain Birbeck granules (see Langerhan Cells, Chap. 17, and discussion of antigen-presenting cells, p. 535). The *myoid cell* is present in the thymus of many species. It is more abundant in human fetuses than in adults. It contains myofilaments and in some species may appear as a well-developed muscle cell. Sarcomeres are not

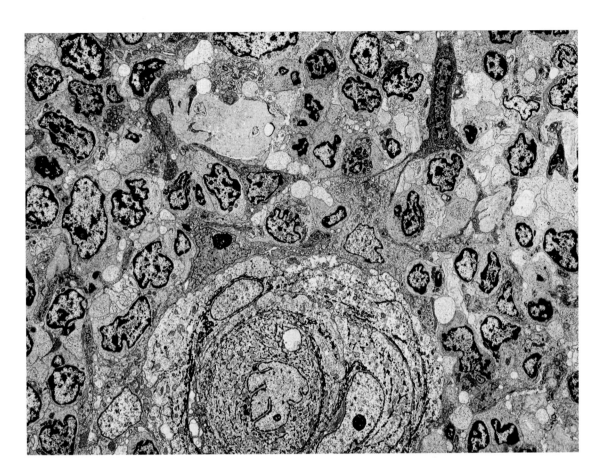

well developed in human beings. Eosinophils and other granulocytes are present in the young thymus; erythroblasts have also been reported. Mast cells may be present in large number in aged thymuses, where they are largely confined to the inner medulla, septae, and capsule. In NZB mice, mast cells may be massively produced within the cortex, presumably from thymic lymphocytes (see below). Plasma cells may occur in the thymus, again largely restricted to surrounding connective tissues but within the parenchyma of the gland as well. Lymphatic nodules may occur pathologically in the thymus. They are restricted to the capsule, septae, and inner medula.

Organization of Parenchyma and Vasculature

The line between the cortex and the medulla of the thymus often appears abrupt. The cortex contains most of the lymphocytes and the medulla contains all of the thymic corpuscles, but both the cortex and the medulla are lymphoepithelial

14–6 Human thymic medulla. There is a large thymic corpuscle along the lower margin. Note the concentric pattern of the epithelial cells and the keratin (dense linear material). The rest of the field consists of branching epithelial cells and lymphocytes and macrophages held within the branches. (From the work of Robert Rouse.)

structures and should be regarded as a continuum. In fact, a simple layer of epithelial cells and their basal lamina runs as a boundary line around both cortex and medulla, thus enclosing both. The connective tissues of the capsule and septae lie outside the lymphoepithelial cortex and medulla, peripheral to the epithelial boundary line (Fig. 14–2). Thymic arteries (branches of the subclavian artery) enter the thymus from the surrounding connective tissues, pass down the septae, and enter the medulla. The vessels that enter the gland and ramify carry in with them a sheath of connective tissue that is continuous with the capsule and septae. As these vessels penetrate the lymphoepithelial cortex and outer medulla (see below), they bring with them a

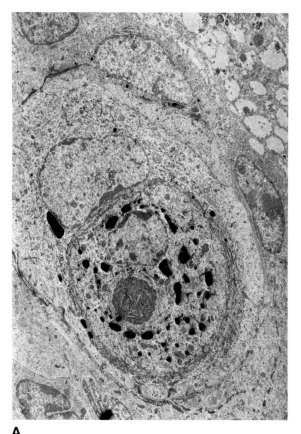

A

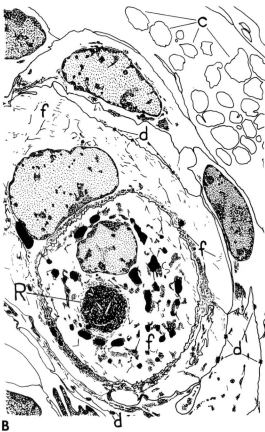

B

14–7 Thymus of a guinea pig. **A.** Electron micrograph of a thymic corpuscle. There is a small compressed central cell (labeled R in the accompanying tracing). Note the concentric pattern of the cells. The inner cells have droplets, probably keratohyaline droplets. Cytoplasmic filaments and desmosomes contribute to this corpuscle. A portion of an epithelial cell in the cytoreticulum in the right upper corner contains intracytoplasmic vacuoles. (From Kohnen, P., and Weiss, L. 1964. Anat. Rec. 148:29 [Fig. 1]). **B.** Tracing of the corpuscle shown in part A. Desmosomes are indicated by **d**, cytoplasmic filaments by **f**, and intracytoplasmic vacuoles by **c**. **R** is degenerated nucleus. × 5,000.

layer of epithelial cells that lies on a basal lamina continuous with the epithelial boundary layer described above (Figs. 14–2 and 14–8 to 14–9). Thus the vessels are surrounded by an epithelial sheath. The connective tissue sheath becomes attenuated as it extends along the smaller ramifications, and is quite slight around the fine cortical vessels. The vascular lumen in the lym-

phoepithelial zones is thereby separated from thymic lymphocytes by a number of layers that are, in order: endothelium (and in arteries and veins, a muscular coat), endothelial basal lamina, perivascular connective tissue, epithelial basal lamina, and epithelium. (See Figs. 14–2, 14–8, and 14–9.) These layers constitute the blood–thymus barrier.

The endothelium of thymic blood vessels and its basal lamina are continuous. There are no high endothelial venules of the sort present in lymph nodes. The connective tissue sheath can be quite thick and cellular around the larger vessels, which enter the gland in the central medulla. In fact, Pereira and Clermont recognize an *inner medulla* that is vascular and made of mesenchymal tissues in distinction to an *outer medulla*, which is lymphoepithelial and enclosed within an epithelial boundary layer. It is within the connective tissue of the inner medulla—and in its extensions throughout the gland as it runs along blood vessels—that many of the plasma cells, granulocytes, mast cells,

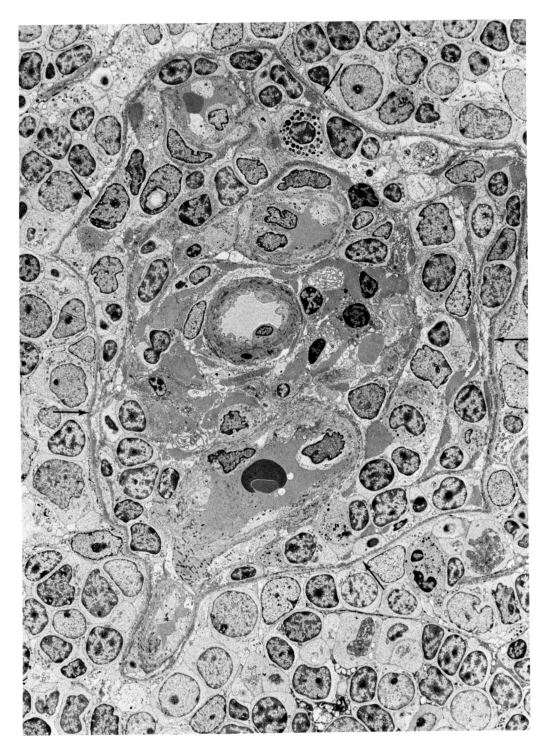

14–8 Human thymus, near the border of the cortex and the medulla. An arteriole with several branches as surrounded by a perivascular connective tissue space limited by epithelial–reticular cells **(arrows).** × 1,850. (From Bearman, R. M., Bensch, K. G., and Levine, G. D. 1975. Anat. Rec. 183:485.) See Fig. 14–6.

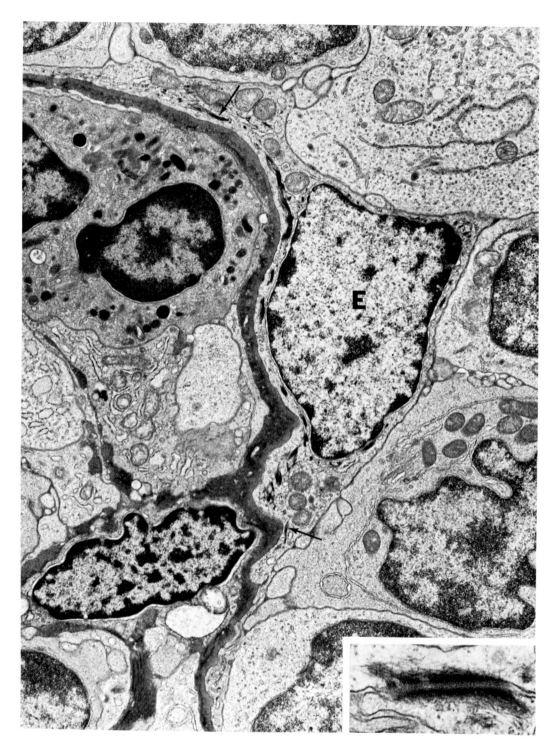

14–9 Human thymus: a higher magnification of the border of the perivascular space and the thymic parenchyma. An epithelial-reticular cell **(E)** delineates the space, which is to the left of the cell. The epithelial-reticular cell contains prominent tonofilaments **(arrows)**. × 16,500. **Inset.** Desmosome between two epithelial-reticular cells. × 50,000 (From Bearman, R.M., Bensch, K.G., and Levine, G. D. 1975. Anat. Rec. 183:485.)

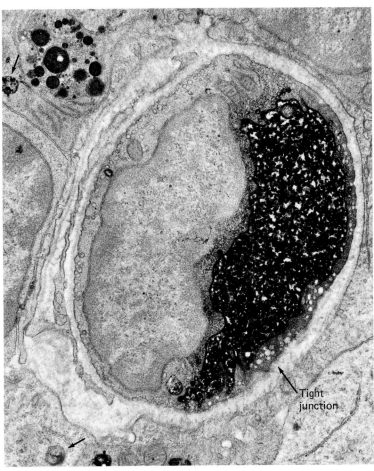

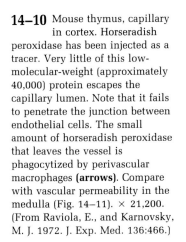

14–10 Mouse thymus, capillary in cortex. Horseradish peroxidase has been injected as a tracer. Very little of this low-molecular-weight (approximately 40,000) protein escapes the capillary lumen. Note that it fails to penetrate the junction between endothelial cells. The small amount of horseradish peroxidase that leaves the vessel is phagocytized by perivascular macrophages **(arrows)**. Compare with vascular permeability in the medulla (Fig. 14–11). × 21,200. (From Raviola, E., and Karnovsky, M. J. 1972. J. Exp. Med. 136:466.)

macrophages, and other connective-tissue cell types are concentrated. The inner medulla is laced with reticular fibers and contains a mesenchymal reticulum in contrast to the cytoreticulum of the lymphoepithelial portion of the thymus. Levine and Bearman recognize epithelial and mesenchymal components of the thymus. They define an *intraparenchymal compartment* (IPC) composed of lymphoepithelial cortex and medulla and an *extraparenchymal compartment* (EPC) composed of blood vessels and surrounding connective tissue. The epithelial boundary layer with its basal lamina described above excludes the EPC. It is, in fact, the border of the IPC and is continuous with the subcapsular epithelial border around the perimeter of the gland.

A *blood–thymus barrier* exists that is impervious to such particulate and protein tracers as lanthanum, ferritin, and horseradish peroxidase. The epithelial cell layer surrounding the vasculature is evidently a major element in this barrier. Raviola and Karnovsky have described the barrier as tight in most of the cortex but leaky in the juxtamedullary cortex (Figs. 14–10 and 14–11). Pereira and Clermont, however, have found the barrier to be tight throughout the thymus, except in the inner medulla.

The major blood vessels branch from the medulla and the corticomedullary junction. Slender arterial vessels run high in the cortex, breaking into capillaries beneath the capsule. Venules run back toward the corticomedullary junction and drain into veins there or in the inner medulla. The stem cells of T lymphocytes probably come into the gland through blood vessels and leave the vasculature beneath the capsule, selectively crossing the blood–thymus barrier and entering the intraparenchymal compartment high in the cortex. There they begin to proliferate and differentiate into T cells, which move deeper into the gland toward the corticomedullary junction.

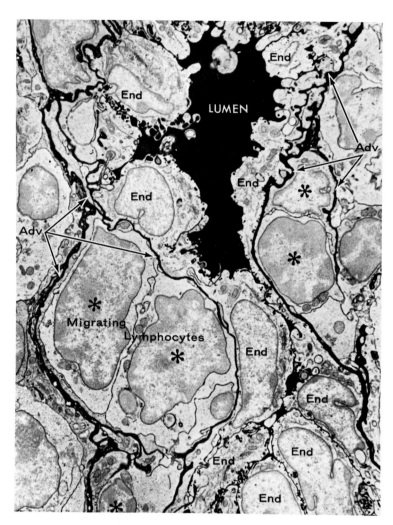

14-11 Mouse thymus, venule in medulla. Horseradish peroxidase has been injected as a tracer. In less than 5 min there has been an impressive leakage, staining the epithelial basal lamina and the adventitia **(Adv)** with the same intensity as the plasma in the lumen of the vessel. Note the irregular endothelium **(End)** bearing many pinocytotic vesicles containing the peroxidase tracer. The thick connective tissue adventitial layer **(Adv)** is traversed by migrating lymphocytes **(asterisks)** which are probably moving toward the lumen and into the circulation. Compare with Fig. 14-10. × 7,100. (From Raviola, E., and Karnovsky, M. J. 1972. J. Exp. Med. 136:466.)

Lymphatic Vessels. Efferent lymphatic vessels lie in the inner medulla of the thymus, run through septae and drain into mediastinal lymph nodes. They, as do veins, carry T lymphocytes from the thymus. There appear to be no afferent lymphatic vessels.

Nerve Supply. The capsule of the thymus is moderately rich in small myelinated and unmyelinated nerves from the vagus, cardiac plexus, first thoracic ganglion, and ansa hypoglossi. Vasomotor nerves enter the organ alongside its blood vessels.

Development

The human thymus develops bilaterally from the third branchial pouches. There may be small contributions from the fourth. The thymic rudi-

ment in embryos of 10-mm crown–rump length (CRL) is a slender, tubular prolongation of branchial epithelium which extends caudad and mediad. The epithelium is of endodermal origin, but it is likely that an ectodermal contribution occurs. There may also be a contribution from the neural crest. The rudiment reaches into the mediastinum just caudal to the thyroid and parathyroid rudiments. The tip of the thymic prolongation proliferates, becoming bulbous. The intermediate portion, constituting the connection to the pharynx, vanishes and leaves the proliferating terminal bulb free in the mediastinum at 35-mm CRL. The epithelial rudiment becomes surrounded by a layer of mesenchyme. Soon afterwards, lymphocyte stem cells penetrate the mesenchyme, enter the epithelium, and lymphocytes and epithelial cells proliferate. The lobular pattern of the thymus becomes evident at

40-mm CRL. Thymic corpuscles appear at 60 to 70 mm.

The development of the thymus outstrips that of the remaining lymphatic organs. Whereas the thymus is rather fully developed prenatally, the spleen and lymph nodes are not.

The thymus may fail to develop normally. Defective thymic development in human beings is found in the Di George syndrome and Swiss-type agammaglobulinemia. A valuable animal model in which the thymus fails to develop normally is the nude (nu/nu) mutant mouse.

Involution

Involution, the process of atrophy and depletion, is related to age. After puberty the thymus gradually decreases in weight and suffers a considerable loss of cortical lymphocytes and of epithelial cells, both of which are replaced by fat.

Table 14–1 Age and Thymus Weight

Age, years	Weight, g
Newborn	13.26
1–5	22.98
6–10	26.10
11–15	37.52
16–20	25.58
21–25	24.73
26–35	19.87
36–45	16.27
46–55	12.85
56–65	16.08
66–75	6.00

There is a decrease in the number of the thymic corpuscles but an increase in their size. The septae show a proportionate increase in width as the lobules atrophy (Table 14–1 and Figs. 14–1 and 14–12).

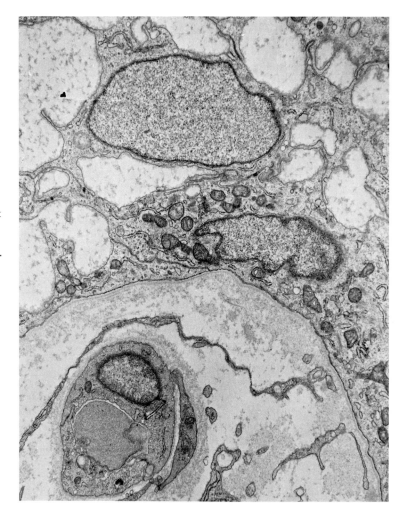

14–12 Human thymic cortex involution. A capillary at the bottom of the field lies in a perivascular space and is surrounded by an atrophic cortex. Lymphocytes have dropped out and the epithelial-reticular cells that remain form a fluid-filled meshwork. × 1,700. (From the work of G. D. Levine.)

Normal age-associated involution of the thymus should not be unduly emphasized, however, since the organ remains substantive and functional even in late adulthood. On the other hand, involution induced by stress may be severe and sudden. Such stress or accidental involution is caused by cortisone and related steroid hormones. The circulating levels of these hormones are increased in stress, and they have a lytic effect on immature T lymphocytes in the thymus. Stress involution is characterized by extensive cortical lymphocyte death and phagocytosis. The thymus in infants who die suddenly may be large and has been considered a cause of death, a condition called *status thymolymphaticus*. However, the thymus in this condition is a normal organ and is undiminished by stress involution.

Comparative Anatomy

Thymic tissue is present in every vertebrate. In lower forms it remains associated with the branchial arches, failing to move caudad. In mammals thymuses are remarkably alike, although differences in the development of thymic corpuscles, myoid cells, cysts, and other such structures may be found.

Functions of the Thymus

T-Lymphocyte Production

The thymus receives stem cells from the bone marrow (and from fetal liver before the marrow develops) and provides the microenvironment for them to develop into immunologically competent T cells. These T cells are released to undergo final maturation in the spleen and then begin a long life circulating and recirculating through blood and lymph, slowly passing through T-cell zones in peripheral lymphatic tissues. A large component of spleen and lymph nodes consists of T cells, and after neonatal thymectomy, these organs fail to develop fully (Fig. 14–13). The level of small lymphocytes circulating in the blood may be reduced by 60% or more; that in thoracic duct lymph may be reduced to an even lower level. The differentiation and migrations of T cells and their functions are discussed under Lymphocytes in Chaps. 11, 12, 15, and 16.

Thymectomy (or congenital athymia) results in severe immunological defects due primarily to a deficiency of T cells, if the operation is performed in the neonatal period before the thymus is able to carry out large-scale seeding of peripheral lymphatic organs with T cells (Fig. 14–13). Cellular immunity is impaired. Thus, after thymectomy in the newborn, homografts (a graft from a genetically different animal but one within the same species, as mouse to mouse) may persist indefinitely instead of being rejected within a week or two. Interference also occurs with antibody production against antigens that depend on cooperation of T cells with B cells. These deficiencies can be fully corrected with thymic grafts.

Thymectomy in adults causes no such clearcut changes because the extrathymic lymphatic tissues and circulation are already stocked with T cells. The weight of spleen and lymph nodes is significantly reduced after thymectomy in adult rats, but 6 to 8 weeks are required for the change to develop. However, if adult rats are thymectomized and then irradiated to deplete stores of T cells in their lymphatic tissues, a condition emerges similar to that of the neonate after thymectomy.

Humoral Factors

The thymus secretes a number of immunological regulatory factors whose presence was first deduced from experiments involving neonatal thymectomy. As discussed above, a newborn mouse thymectomized at birth becomes deficient in both lymphocytes and immunological capacity. If a thymus wrapped in a cell-tight filter is inserted into the peritoneal cavity of such a mouse, the animal will have partial restoration of lymphocytes and suffer no immunological deficiencies. Factors appear to diffuse through the wrapping and largely substitute for the thymus. Further support for thymic humoral factors comes from experiments in which immunological competence is restored in thymectomized immunologically deficient female mice when they become pregnant, even though the placenta does not permit cells to move from fetus to mother. The best characterized of thymic humoral factors is *thymosin*, which may be separated into low-molecular-weight glycoprotein fractions (3,100 and 5,250 daltons). Thymosin restores T-cell deficiencies in thymectomized mice, thereby substituting for a thymus. Thymosin has been demonstrated in thymic epithelial cells by immunocytochemistry and is presumably se-

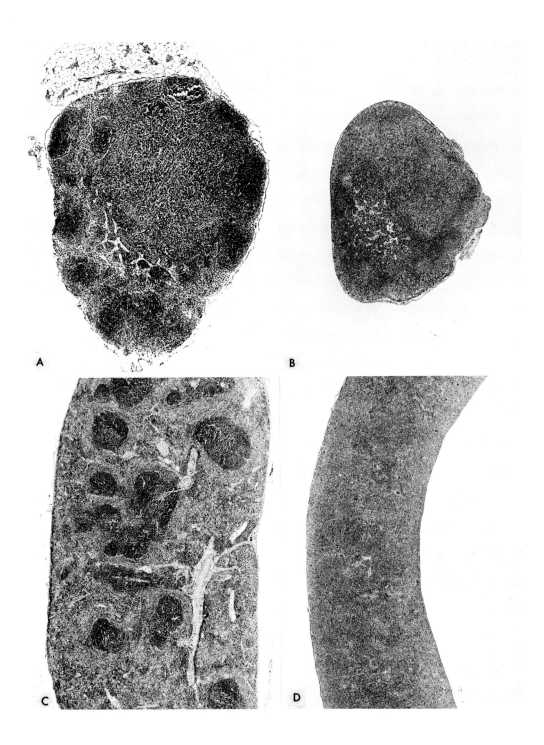

14–13 This plate illustrates the dependence of the lymph nodes and spleen on the thymus. The tissues are taken from C57BL mice. **A.** Lymph node of 8-week-old mouse sham-operated at birth. ×32. **B.** Lymph node of 8-week-old mouse thymectomized at birth. ×32. **C.** Spleen of 7-week-old mouse sham-operated at birth. ×32. **D.** Spleen of 7-week-old mouse thymectomized at birth. ×32. Thymectomy is followed by a decrease in size of the lymph nodes and spleen, due primarily to depletion of small lymphocytes (T cells). (From the work of J. F. A. P. Miller.)

creted by them. *Thymopoietin* (5500d) induces T cell maturation. *Thymic humoral factor* enhances the graft vs. host reaction. The *serum thymic factor* (847d) induces the development of markers in T cells. Secretion of a factor mitogenic for developing T cells has been ascribed to the thymic macrophages, a function related to the production of granulocyte colony stimulating factors (CSF-G) by macrophages (see Chap. 12).

Major Histocompatibility Complex Antigens

Epithelial-reticular cells, lymphocytes, and, indeed, virtually every cell in the body express an array of MHC antigens on their surface distinctive to cell type and development. These antigens are gene products whose background is as follows: There is a "supergene" known as the *major histocompatibility gene complex (MHC)*. It is on chromosome 17 in mice and chromosome 6 in human beings. The MHC complex is called the H-2 system in mice and the HLA (histocompatibility linked antigens) system in human beings. This supergene is subdivided into four major subdivisions: K, I, S, and D; each of them is subdivided so that, for example, subregions of the I region are Ia and Ib. The MHC contains genes that direct the production (through the usual processes of transcription, translation, and protein synthesis) of gene products, which may move to a position on the cell surface or be released to the extracellular environment. Through such gene products the MHC controls a number of immunological functions; and it is possible to correlate the activity of a given MHC subregion with a given immunological function. For example, the genes of the I region control a variety of phenomena associated with cellular recognition as well as with recognition of antigenic foreignness. Mouse T cells that help B cells (T_H or helper T cells) bear surface determinants coded in the Ia region and cytotoxic T cells (T_s or suppressor T cells) have cell-surface determinants coded in the K or D region. Similar arrangements occur in human beings and in other species tested. Rouse et al. and others have found that in the thymus the epithelial-reticular cells, which are intimately associated with developing T cells, have MHC gene products on their surfaces. The gene products of different regions of the MHC complex, moreover, are expressed in different patterns on the thymic cytoreticulum formed by the epithelial-reticular cells. The gene products of the Ia region are present throughout the thymic cortex, whereas those of the rest of the I region and of the K and D regions are expressed only variably. Thus, developing T lymphocytes are exposed, during their intimate association with epithelial-reticular cells, to a highly specific gene product expressing self. This exposure may well be a factor in determining which T cells are induced to divide and be released (those that recognize and react against foreign materials or nonself) and which are destroyed or not permitted to proliferate (those that would react against self and induce autoimmune disease). Monoclonal antibodies may be prepared against MHC antigens and, when coupled to horseradish peroxidase or another marker, may be used as the basis of a cytochemical test for demonstrating MHC antigens in tissue section (Fig. 14–14).

Mast Cell and Eosinophil Differentiation

Mast cells may be present within the thymus; in certain strains of mice, such as the NZB, they are present in massive numbers. In tissue culture of thymus, Ginsburg and Sachs showed large-scale differentiation of mast cells from thymic lymphocytes. The Ishizakas demonstrated that IgE receptors appeared on the surface of these cells at about the time cytoplasmic granules began to appear in their cytoplasm. Moreover, the thymic cells undergoing transformation into mast cells, were not T cells. Therefore, the thymus contains stem cells for mast cell differentiation.

The thymus is necessary for heightened eosinophilopoiesis. Nude mice and thymectomized animals have normal basal levels of eosinophils but are unable to produce increased numbers after such stimuli as infection with helminths.

Bursa of Fabricius

The bursa of Fabricius is a cloacal lymphoepithelial organ in birds that receives stem cells from bone marrow and induces them to differentiate into B cells. It is analogous to that other gut-derived lymphoepithelial organ, the thymus, which receives stem cells from the bone marrow and induces their differentiation into T cells. The letters T and B are taken from Thymus and Bursa.

The bursa originates as an epithelial diverticulum of the cloaca and becomes infiltrated by immigrated lymphocytes. In the bursa, the epithelial diverticulum retains connection with the cloaca and forms follicles around which the lymphocytes are organized. The bursa involutes markedly on sexual maturation. In fact, its development may be entirely suppressed by applying male sex hormones to the shell of embryonated eggs. In mammals, the bursal equivalent appears to be bone marrow.

References and Selected Bibliography

General

Bearman, R. M., Levine, G. D., and Bensch, K. G. 1978. The ultrastructure of the normal human thymus. Anat. Rec. 190:755.

Chapman, W. L., Jr., and Allen, J. R. 1971. The fine structure of the thymus of the fetal and neonatal monkey (Macaca mulatta). Z. Zellforsch. Mikrosk. Anat. 114:220.

Clark, S. L., Jr. 1973. The intrathymic environment. In A. J. S. Davies and R. L. Carter (eds.), Contemporary Topics in Immunobiology, Vol. 2, Thymus Dependency. New York: Plenum Press, p. 77.

Defendi, V., and Metcalf, D. (eds.). 1964. The Thymus. Philadelphia: Wistar Institute Press.

Hwang, W. S., Ho, T. Y., Luk, S. C., and Simon, G. T. 1974. Ultrastructure of the rat thymus. A transmission, scanning electron microscope, and morphometric study. Lab. Invest. 31:473.

Janossy, G., Thomas, J. A., Bollum, F. J., et al. 1980. The human thymic microenvironment: An immunohistological study. J. Immunol. 125:202.

Kendall, M. D. (ed.). 1981. The Thymus Gland. Academic Press. London.

Kindred, J. E. 1940. A quantitative study of the hematopoietic organs of young albino rats. Am. J. Anat. 67:99.

Kohnen, P., and Weiss, L. 1964. An electron microscopic study of thymic corpuscles in the guinea pig and the mouse. Anat. Rec. 148:29.

Parrott, D. M. V., De Sousa, M. A. B., and East, J. 1966. Thymus-dependent areas in the lymphoid areas of neonatally thymectomized mice. J. Exp. Med. 123:191.

Pereira, G., and Clermont, Y. 1971. Distribution of cell web-containing epithelial reticular cells in the rat thymus. Anat. Rec. 169:613.

Porter, R., and Whelan, J. 1981. Microenvironments in hematopoietic and lymphoid differentiation. Ciba Foundation Symposium 84. London: Pitman.

van Haelst, U. J. G. 1967. Light and electron microscopic study of the normal and pathological thymus of the rat. I. The normal thymus. Z. Zellforsch. Mikrosk. Anat. 77:534.

van Haelst, U. J. G. 1969. Light and electron microscopic study of the normal and pathological thymus of the rat. III. A mesenchymal histiocytic type of cell. Z. Zellforsch. Mikrosk. Anat. 99:198.

Cellular Migration

Harris, J. E., and Ford, C. E. 1964. Cellular traffic of the thymus: Experiments with chromosome markers. I. Evidence that the thymus plays an instructional part. Nature (Lond.) 201:884.

Harris, J. E., Ford, C. E., Barnes, D. W. H., and Evans, E. P. 1964. Cellular traffic of the thymus: Experiments with chromosome markers. II. Evidence from parabiosis for an afferent stream of cells. Nature (Lond.) 201:886.

Linna, J., and Stillstrom, J. 1966. Migration of cells from the thymus to the spleen in young guinea pigs. Acta Pathol. Microbiol. Scand. 68:465.

Sainte-Marie, G., and Peng, F. S. 1971. Emigration of thymocytes from the thymus. A review and study of the problem. Rev. Can. Biol. 30:51.

Toro, I., and Olah, I. 1967. Penetration of thymocytes into the blood circulation. J. Ultrastruct. Res. 17:439.

Weissman, I. L. 1967. Thymus cell migration. J. Exp. Med. 126:291.

Development and Regeneration

Downey, H. 1948. Cytology of rabbit thymus and regeneration of its thymocytes after irradiation, with some notes on the human thymus. Blood 3:1315.

Haar, J. L. 1974. Light and electron microscopy of the human fetal thymus. Anat. Rec. 179:463.

Hirokawa, K. 1969. Electron microscopic observation of the human thymus of the fetus and the newborn. Acta Pathol. Jpn. 19:1.

Mandel, T. 1970. Differentiation of epithelial cells in the mouse thymus. Z. Zellforsch. Mikrosk. Anat. 106:498.

Moore, M. A. S., and Owen, J. J. T. 1967. Experimental studies on the development of the thymus. J. Exp. Med. 126:715.

Immunological Role

Aranson, B. G., and Wennersten, C. 1962. Role of the thymus in immune reaction in rats. II. Suppressive effect of thymectomy at birth on reactions of delayed (cellular) hypersensitivity and the circulating small lymphocyte. J. Exp. Med. 116:177.

Jankovic, B., Waksman, B. H., and Aranson, B. G. 1962. Role of the thymus in immune reactions in rats. I. The immunologic response to bovine serum albumin (antibody formation, arthus reactivity and delayed hypersensitivity) in rats thymectomized or splenectomized at various times after birth. J. Exp. Med. 116:159.

Metcalf, D. 1966. The thymus: Its role in immune responses, leukaemia development and carcinogenesis. In Recent Results in Cancer Research, Vol. 5. Berlin: Springer-Verlag OHG.

Miller, J. F. A. P. 1962. Effect of neonatal thymectomy on the immunological responsiveness of the mouse. Proc. R. Soc. Lond. (Biol.) 156:415.

Waksman, B. H., Aranson, B. G., and Jankovic, B. D. 1962. Role of the thymus in immune reactions in rats. III. Changes in the lymphoid organs of thymectomized rats. J. Exp. Med. 116:187.

Mast Cells

Ginsburg, H., and Sachs, L. 1963. Formation of pure suspensions of mast cells in tissue culture by differentiation of lymphoid cells from the mouse thymus. J. Natl. Cancer Inst. 31:1.

Ishizaka, T., Okadaira, H., Mauser, L. E., and Ishizaka, K. 1976. Development of rat mast cells in vitro. I. Differentiation of mast cells from thymus cells. J. Immunol. 116:747.

MHC Antigens

Rouse, R. V., van Ewijk, W., Jones, P. P., and Weissman, I. L. 1979. Expression of MHC antigens by mouse thymic dendritic cells. J. Immunol. 122:2508.

van Ewijk, W., Rouse, R. V., and Weissan, I. L. 1980. Distribution of H-2 microenvironments in the mouse thymus. J. Histochem. Cytochem. 28:1089.

Pathology

Levine, G. D., Rosai, J., Bearman, R. M., and Polliack, A. 1975. The fine structure of thymoma, with emphasis on its differential diagnosis. A study of 10 cases. Am. J. Pathol. 81:49.

Rosai, J., and Levine, G. D. 1975. Tumors of the Thymus, 2nd Ser., Atlas of Tumor Pathology. Washington, D. C.: Armed Forces Institute of Pathology.

Wolstenholme, G. E. W., and Porter, R. (eds.). 1966. The Thymus: Experimental and Clinical Studies, a Ciba Foundation Symposium. Boston: Little, Brown and Company.

T Cells

Bevan, M. J., and Fink, P. J. 1978. The influence of thymus H-2 antigens on the specificity of maturing killer and helper cells. Immunol. Rev. 42:3.

Scollay, R., Jacobs, S., Jerabek, L., Butcher, E., and Weissman, I. 1980. T cell maturation: Thymocyte and thymus migrant subpopulations defined with monoclonal antibodies to MHC region antigens. J. Immunol. 124:2845.

Takatsu, K., and Ishizaka, K. 1976. Reagenic antibody formation in the mouse: VIII. Depression of the ongoing IgE antibody formation by suppressor T-cells. J. Immunol. 117:1211.

Thymic Humoral Factors

Bach, J.-F., and Papiernik, M. 1981. Cellular and molecular signals in T-cell differentiation. In Ciba Foundation Symposium 84. Microenvironments in haemopoietic and lymphoid differentiation. Porter, R., and Whelan, I. (eds.). Pitman, p. 215.

Levey, R. H., Trainin, N., and Law, L. W. 1963. Evidence for function of thymic tissue in diffusion chambers implanted in neonatally thymectomized mice. J. Natl. Cancer Inst. 31:199.

Osoba, D., and Miller, J. F. A. P. 1964. The lymphoid tissues and immune responses to neonatally thymectomized mice bearing thymic tissues in millipore diffusion chambers. J. Exp. Med. 119:177.

Vasculature

Bearman, R. M., Bensch, K. G., and Levine, G. D. 1975. The normal human thymic vasculature: An ultrastructural study. Anat. Rec. 183:485.

Raviola, E., and Karnovsky, M. J. 1972. Evidence for a blood–thymus barrier using electron-opaque tracers. J. Exp. Med. 136:466.

Bursa of Fabricius

Jolly, J. 1915. La bourse de Fabricius et les organes lympho-épithéliaux. Arch. Anat. Microbiol. 16:363.

Moore, M. A. S., and Owen, J. J. T. 1966. Experimental studies on the development of the bursa of Fabricius. Dev. Biol. 14:40.

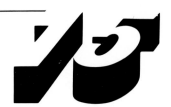

Lymphatic Vessels and Lymph Nodes

Leon Weiss

Lymphatic Vessels

Lymphatic vessels originate in connective tissue spaces as anastomosing capillaries. The capillaries flow into larger *collecting vessels;* the largest and most proximal empty into veins in the base of the neck as the left and right thoracic ducts. Like blood vessels, lymphatic vessels are an arborized system of endothelial-lined tubes that carry cellular elements suspended in a fluid intercellular substance. Unlike blood vessels, they do not form a circular system but carry their contents, called *lymph,* in only one direction, toward the base of the neck. Lymphatic vessels recover fluids that escape into the connective tissue spaces from blood capillaries and venules and return them to the blood. In mammals, dense encapsulated collections of lymphocytes called *lymph nodes* lie across lymphatic vessels, and lymph percolates through them. Lymph nodes filter lymph and serve as stations for traffic of T and B cells and their immunological activities.

Distribution

Lymphatic capillaries are most numerous beneath body surfaces: the skin; the mucous membranes of the gastrointestinal, respiratory, and genitourinary tracts; and subserous tissues. Lymphatic capillaries may be arranged in superficial and deep plexuses (Figs. 15–1 to 15–3), each of which is deeper than blood capillaries. Parts of the body are not supplied with lymphatics. The central nervous system, globus oculi, and the

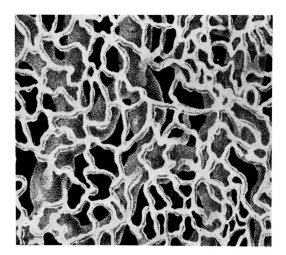

15–1 Lymphatic vessels of a dog. Superficial and deep vessels in the wall of the stomach as viewed from the surface. × 30. (From Teichmann.)

15–2 Lymphatic network in the human appendix as viewed from the surface. Note the enlargement of vessels over the lymphoid nodules and in the valves in the larger vessels. × 40. (From Teichmann.)

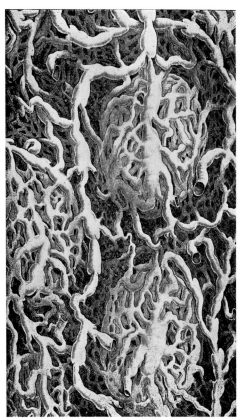

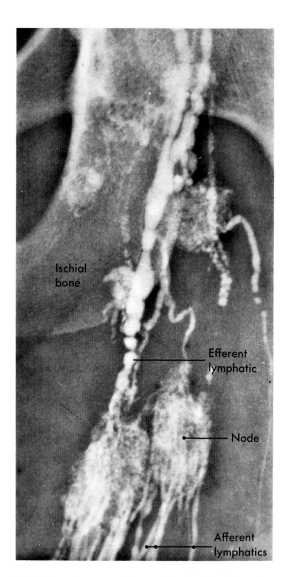

15–3 Lymphogram of human inguinal lymph nodes and lymphatics. A radiopaque dye injected into the lymphatic vessels in the thigh is carried by afferent lymphatic vessels into the draining lymph nodes of the inguinal region. The dye flows through the nodes and enters its efferent lymphatic vessels. The dye will continue centrally through the lymphatic system and eventually flow into the veins at the base of the neck. This lymphogram is an x-ray of the inguinal region several minutes after the injection of dye. Against the background of the soft tissues of the thigh and the pelvic bones, the lymphatic vessels and nodes are seen. Note the large number of slender afferent lymphatics. The nodes are oval, the dark zones within them representing lymphocytes and other cells around which the dye flows. The efferent lymphatics have a wide caliber. The beaded appearance of the largest vessel is due to the presence of valves.

bone marrow contain none. Striated (noncardiac) muscles contain lymphatic vessels only in the perimysium. Within the liver, lymphatic capillaries reach into the perilobular spaces and do not extend into the liver lobule. Loci in the liver, spleen, and bone marrow that are supplied by venous sinusoids lack lymphatics. The sinusoids appear to subserve functions of lymphatic vessels.

Structure

Lymphatic capillaries may reach 100 μm in diameter. Their walls are made of flattened endothelium (Figs. 15–4 to 15–6). Endothelial cells are attached to one another along their perimeter by zonulae adhaerens, and contiguous cells may overlap in flap-like fashion. The endothelium forms a complete layer but in some cases, such as in the lacteals of the intestinal villi, small apertures are present. The basement membrane is poorly developed. Fine *anchoring filaments* run from perivascular bundles of collagen and attach

15–4 Skin of guinea pig. A lymphatic capillary is present in the dermis. A small blood-filled venule is nearby. (From D. Chou and L. Weiss, in Weiss, L. 1972. Cells and Tissues of the Immune System. Englewood Cliffs, N.J.: Prentice-Hall, Inc.)

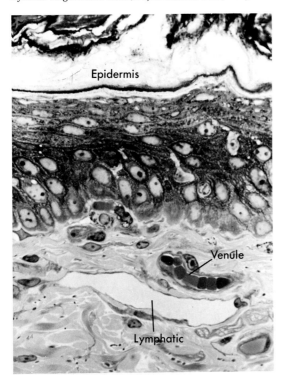

to the outer surface of the endothelium. In inflammation, the pressure on perilymphatic tissues increases, but the anchoring filaments pull on the lymphatic vessel wall like a guy rope on a tent and help keep the vessel open (see Fig. 15–5). *Collecting vessels* are structurally similar to veins but without definite layers. Like the pattern seen in blood vessels, three coats or tunics are present: *intima, media,* and *adventitia* (Fig. 15–7). Even in the largest and best-developed lymphatic vessel, the left *thoracic duct,* it is difficult to delineate these layers. This thoracic duct, 4 to 6 μm in diameter, has an internal elastic membrane and is supplied by blood vessels and nerves that penetrate its adventitia and media, as do vasa vasorum and nerves of blood vessels.

Collecting vessels contain valves (Figs. 15–3 and 15–7), paired cusps each originating from opposite endothelial surfaces and extending into the lumen. The base of a single valve cusp takes up approximately 180° of circumference, so that the entire circumference of the vessel wall provides attachment for a valve. Occasional tricuspid valves are found. Cusps are formed as folds of endothelium. A few connective tissue fibers and even muscle fibers extend between the folded endothelial surfaces of the cusps from the subendothelial tissue. The cusps project in the direction of lymph flow and prevent back-flow. A valve in each of the great lymphatic channels at its junction with the systemic veins prevents the gurgitation of blood into the lymphatic system. Valves are responsible for the beaded appearance of lymphatic vessels; the vessel is constricted at the attachment of the base of the valve and dilated beyond.

Lymphatic vessels anastomose with one another and tend to travel in company with blood vessels (usually veins), which may be girdled by lymphatics. Lymph is carried to lymph nodes by afferent lymphatic vessels and from them by efferent vessels (Figs. 15–3). It is likely that no lymph reaches venous blood without flowing through at least one node.

Function

Lymphatic vessels return to the blood material that has escaped blood vessels. The walls of blood capillaries and venules are semipermeable membranes that permit the diffusion of small-molecular-weight materials through them and retain larger molecules (such as proteins and fatty complexes) and the cellular elements of the

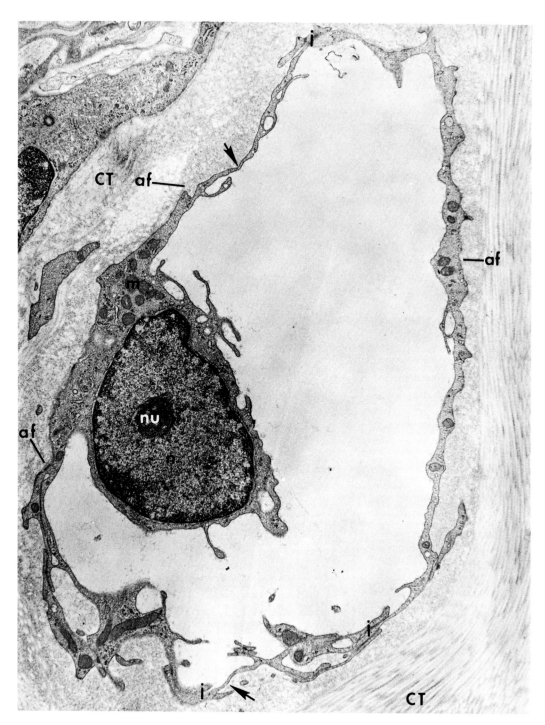

15–5 Cross section of lymphatic capillary. A close association of the surrounding interstitial elements **(CT)** with the capillary wall is maintained by numerous anchoring filaments **(af),** which appear as a network of small filaments in this low-power micrograph. The extreme attenuations **(arrows)** achieved by the endothelium are illustrated in various regions of the capillary wall. The nucleus **(n)** with its nucleolus **(nu)** protrudes into the lumen, and several intercellular junctions **(i)** are observed. Mitochondria **(m)** occur in the perinuclear regions and also throughout the thin cytoplasmic rim of the endothelial wall. × 11,000. (From the work of L. Leak and J. Burke.)

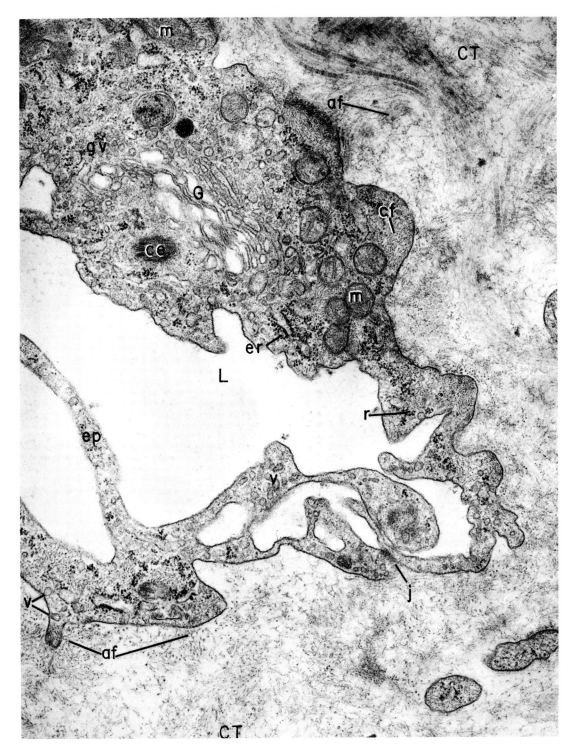

15–6 Lymphatic capillary. In this electron micrograph, the wall of the lymphatic capillary lies in its connective tissue bed. The lymphatic endothelium contains mitochondria **(m)**, a Golgi complex **(G)**, Golgi vesicles **(gv)**, ribosomes **(r)**, rough ER **(er)**, a centriole **(ce)**, luminal endothelial processes **(ep)**, and pinocytotic vesicles **(v)**. Anchoring filaments **(af)** are present. **L**, lumen; **CT**, connective tissue; **j**, junction complex of endothelial cells. (From the work of L. Leak and J. Burke.)

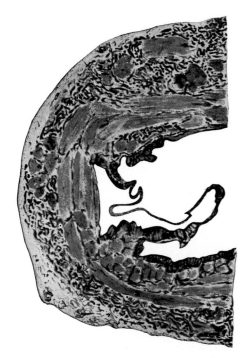

15–7 Lumbar lymphatic trunk of a human adult. A valve is present. Weigert's resorcinfuchsin and picroindigo carmine stain. (From the work of Kajava.)

blood. Small but cumulatively significant amounts of plasma protein do escape from blood vessels, however, with large volumes of fluid. The bathing of perivascular connective tissues by this transudate constitutes an essential physiological process. This is the means by which hormones, antibodies, enzymes and other macromolecules, low-molecular-weight molecules, and fluids reach the cells and intercellular matrix of the body. At least a part of this protein-containing fluid is absorbed into lymphatic capillaries and carried back to the blood. The importance of conserving plasma protein is shown by the following case report from Crandall, et al. (1943).

A 30-year-old woman was shot in the left side of the neck, 1 hour before admission to the hospital. The left jugular vein was ligated 2 days after admission. During the operation straw-colored fluid steadily welled up in the wound so that the skin was not closed. After the operation the dressings were rapidly saturated with this fluid and, for the next 6 weeks, a ceaseless leakage of what was unquestionably thoracic duct lymph continued. The patient at once took the regular hospital diet; after she had eaten, the leaking fluid became milky. But she lost weight at the rate of 5 lb. a week

and her plasma protein fell to 3.5 gm per 100 ml in just a month. A diet high in protein brought this to 4.6 gm per 100 ml in 13 days, but weight loss continued. Accordingly, in a second operation the thoracic duct was ligated and the wound closed. For 2 weeks after this ligation, the patient had cramps after eating but she gained 16 lb. in a month and was discharged free of complaints. The concentration of protein in the lymph ranged from 3.19 to 5.28 per 100 ml.

As suggested by the above report, lymphatic vessels absorb fat, especially neutral fat, from the intestine. The patient ingested olive oil stained with Sudan IV. Approximately 90 min after she swallowed the labeled olive oil, the dye appeared in thoracic duct lymph. In the resting state, probably 95% of the volume of thoracic duct lymph comes from the liver and intestine. Most of the protein in thoracic duct lymph originates in the liver.

There is a small but significant loss of cells from the blood (including red blood cells). Most of these cells function and are lost in the perivascular tissue. Some are picked up by lymphatics and returned to the blood. In addition, there is regular traffic of fluid and cells, especially macrophages, from serosal cavities (such as the peritoneal, and pericardial) via lymph into blood.

The permeability of lymphatic vessels increases greatly under certain mild conditions that occur normally or that represent at most, only a slight departure from the normal. Pressure sufficient to obstruct the flow of lymph causes permeability to increase before visible dilation of the lymphatic occurs. Stroking the skin with a blunt wire or scratching the skin without breaking the epidermis causes an immediate great increase in lymphatic permeability. Warming the ears of mice to 43°C increases permeability. Histamine also heightens lymphatic permeability. Particles and fluids cross the lymphatic endothelium by transcytosis, as is also characteristic of the endothelium of blood vessels (see Chap. 9). Cells cross through interendothelial-cell junctions.

Larger lymphatic vessels are supplied by vasomotor nerves and respond to such powerful constrictor agents as epinephrine or pituitrin. Lymphatic capillaries probably do not respond. They are, however, highly elastic, distensible by one-third without rupture. The flow of lymph is promoted by remitting compression of lymphatic vessels by surrounding structures (particularly muscles and pulsating blood vessels), respiratory movements, propulsive actions of the lymphatic walls (by smooth muscle), and the force of gravity (in the lymphatics above the thoracic duct). The direction of flow is controlled by valves. The rate of flow varies considerably. Trypan blue injected into the hind foot of a dog reaches thoracic duct lymph in seconds. The volume of lymph entering the blood stream from the thoracic duct in resting human subjects averages 1.38 ml per kg per h (range: 3.9–0.38). Flow is increased by ingesting food or water or by abdominal massage.

Lymph Nodes

Lymph nodes are ovoid encapsulated filters of lymph ranging from a few millimeters to more than a centimeter in their largest dimension (Figs. 15–8 to 15–10). They are best developed in mammals where they lie across collecting lymphatic vessels, and lymph flows through them as it moves toward the junctions of lymphatic vessels and veins. Sites rich in nodes are at the base of the extremities, the neck, retroperitoneum, and mediastinum. In birds, lymph nodes consist of loosely organized lymphatic tissue lying alongside lymphatic vessels. Birds have relatively few such nodes, however, and collections of lymphocytes lie scattered through

the pancreas, liver, kidney and other organs. Fish, amphibia, and reptiles lack lymph nodes.

Structure

A lymph node consists of a *capsule* that encloses lymphocytes and other free cells, which are arranged on a reticulum and supplied by blood and lymphatic vessels and nerves.

The capsule is composed of dense collagenous tissue and some muscle. Its outer surface is convex but contains an indentation, the *hilus*, through which lymphatic vessels leave the node and blood vessels enter. Afferent lymphatic vessels pierce the convex surface of the capsule and empty into the node. Trabeculae project from the inner surface of the capsule into the node.

The reticulum is a delicate meshwork composed, as in the spleen, of reticular fibers and reticular cells. The reticular cells are large branched cells that evidently secrete reticular fibers. The fibers lie on the surface of the reticular cells and form a branching meshwork, the *fibrous reticulum*, which can be selectively stained with silver (argyrophilia) and by the periodic acid Schiff (PAS) reaction.

Lymphocytes are the most numerous of the cells within the reticulum. In the periphery of a node they are closely packed, forming a layer

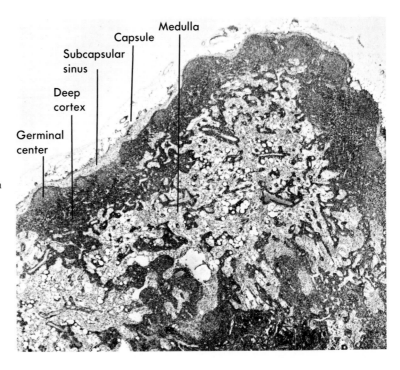

15–8 Human lymph node. Giemsa stain. × 30.

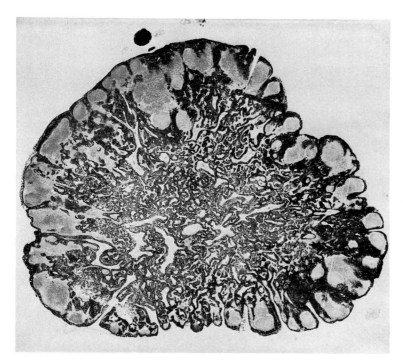

15–9 Lymph node injected with India ink. The sinus system is well outlined. × 10.

15–10 A. Popliteal lymph node of dog; scanning electron micrograph of cut surface of cortex. The capsule is prominent, and trabeculae extend from it into the node. Both the subcapsular sinus and the radial sinuses, which run along the trabeculae, are crisscrossed by the processes of reticular cells and reticular fibers. A germinal center, consisting of compactly organized cells, lies within a lymphatic nodule. × 111. **B.** A higher magnification showing details of capsule, subcapsular sinus, mantle zone of secondary lymphatic nodule and germinal center. × 370. (From Irino, S., Ono, T., Hiraki, K., and Murakami, T. 1974. Blood and Vessel 5:595 [in Japanese].)

A

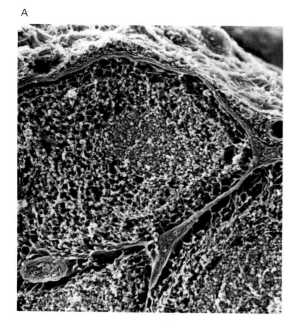

B

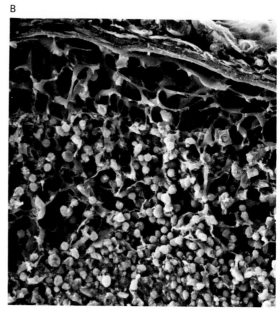

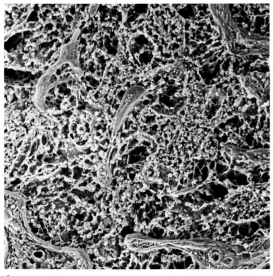

A

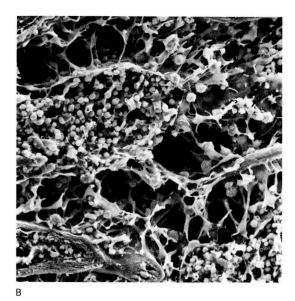

B

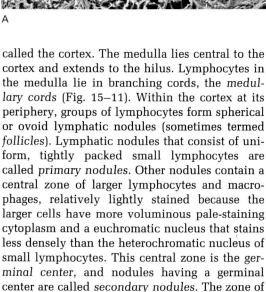

called the cortex. The medulla lies central to the cortex and extends to the hilus. Lymphocytes in the medulla lie in branching cords, the *medullary cords* (Fig. 15–11). Within the cortex at its periphery, groups of lymphocytes form spherical or ovoid lymphatic nodules (sometimes termed *follicles*). Lymphatic nodules that consist of uniform, tightly packed small lymphocytes are called *primary nodules*. Other nodules contain a central zone of larger lymphocytes and macrophages, relatively lightly stained because the larger cells have more voluminous pale-staining cytoplasm and a euchromatic nucleus that stains less densely than the heterochromatic nucleus of small lymphocytes. This central zone is the *germinal center*, and nodules having a germinal center are called *secondary nodules*. The zone of small lymphocytes surrounding the germinal center of the secondary nodule constitutes the *mantle zone*, sometimes termed the *crescent*.

Macrophages are always plentiful throughout lymph nodes and can quickly increase in number as needs arise. Macrophages tend to be most common in the medulla and may occur in large number in germinal centers after antibody formation declines. Macrophages are, of course, phagocytic, but they carry out other functions of secretion, antigen modification, etc., as discussed in Chap. 4.

A system of peripatetic cells has been recognized whose main function appears to be to capture and hold antigen on their surface and to present it to lymphocytes, thereby ensuring an

15–11 **A.** Popliteal lymph node of dog; scanning electron micrograph of cut surface of medulla. Trabeculae lie in the parenchyma, surrounded by lymphatic sinuses whose lumen is crisscrossed by a reticular meshwork. Medullary cords are also present. × 110. **B.** A higher magnification showing a cell-packed medullary cord surrounded by a lymphatic sinus. × 358. (From Irino, S., Ono, T., Hiraki, K., and Murakami, T. 1974. Blood vessel 5:595 [in Japanese].)

immune response. They may also cluster lymphocytes about them. These cells are neither fibroblastic nor phagocytic and are rather large and branched, with ruffled cytoplasmic surfaces. Certain cells in this system may possess a singular cytoplasmic marker known as the *Birbeck granule*.

Antigen presenting cells (APC), which originate in bone marrow, have been seen in many sites in the body and undoubtedly will be found in additional places. In the epidermis a cell long known as the *Langerhans cell* (Chap. 17) has been shown to capture antigen penetrating the skin. The Langerhans cell then moves out of the skin to the regional lymph nodes, carrying the antigen to the lymphocytes there. Langerhans cells, particularly those high in the epidermis, contain Birbeck granules (Chap. 17). An immune response distinctive to the skin, *contact hypersensitivity*, depends upon Langerhans cells. APC lie within the cortex of lymph nodes and the white pulp of the spleen in both B-cell and T-cell zones (see below and Chap. 16). APC in T-cell zones have been referred to as *interdigitating cells*, those in B cell zones as *follicular dendritic cells*. Interdigitating cells have also been observed in the thymus (Chap. 13). Interdigitating cells have Ia antigen of the major histocompatibility complex on their surface, an antigen associated with the capacity to cluster T cells. This capacity appears to facilitate immune responses and to contribute to the development of T cell zones and the phenomena of T-cell homing and sorting.

In addition to the APC of the tissues, there seems to be a cell in this system which travels in blood and lymph. By the usual cytological techniques it is likely identified as a monocyte, but Balfour has identified a rich array of veil-like cytoplasmic surface processes and has termed it the *veil cell*. This cell occasionally shows Birbeck granules. The M cell of the gut epithelium (Chap. 19) may be a candidate for this system of cells.

The presence of lymphatic nodules in the superficial cortex of lymph nodes establishes three cortical zones: (1) the *nodular cortex*; (2) the *internodular cortex*, which lies between nodules; and (3) a *deep* or *tertiary cortex*, which lies below the first two zones and above the medulla. The internodular and teritary cortexes may be taken together as the *diffuse cortex*. B lymphocytes are concentrated in primary nodules and T lymphocytes in the diffuse cortex (see Fig. 15–19). Germinal centers are sites of B-cell differentiation and high-level antibody formation. They are concerned with the development of B memory cells. They also contain T cells and macrophages. Plasma cell formation is initiated there, but few plasma cells are present in germinal centers because as B cells differentiate into plasma cells, they leave germinal centers and move toward the medulla. Medullary cords contain plasma cells, macrophages and lymphocytes, and some granulocytes. They are branching partitions of tissue that extend from the underside of the cortex and converge toward the hilus.

The interactions of the various zones of lymph nodes are discussed below under Immunological Functions.

Vascular Supply

Lymphatic Vessels. Afferent lymphatic vessels, carrying lymph from the connective tissue spaces or from a more peripheral lymph node, pierce the capsule and empty into a large *subcapsular sinus*, which lies directly beneath the capsule and is coextensive with it. *Cortical or radial sinuses* run radially from the subcapsular sinus through the cortex, often along trabeculae. They become *medullary sinuses* as they pass between the medullary cords and converge toward the hilus. There they drain into efferent lymphatic channels.

Lymphatic sinuses are lined by reticular cells, which provide a rather irregular surface that often contains apertures. The lining reticular cells extend cytoplasmic processes that crisscross the lumen (Figs. 15–10 and 15–11), retarding the lymph flow and causing turbulence.

Blood Vessels. Blood vessels enter a node at the hilus. (A few enter at the convex surface of the capsule.) Arterioles reach the cortex through trabeculae and break up into the capillaries, which empty into venules. These venules enter veins that run from cortex to medulla and then leave the node via the hilus. Postcapillary venules lie in the diffuse cortex. They have a cuboidal endothelium and therefore have been called high endothelial venules (HEV). The walls of the HEVs are often infiltrated with small lymphocytes (Figs. 15–12 to 15–18). Gowans and colleagues, using radioactively labeled lymphocytes and autoradiography, showed that these lymphocytes pass from the blood into the parenchyma of the node. They pass between endothelial cells, deeply indenting their lateral plasma membranes. High endothelial venules represent a major pathway by which small lymphocytes, both T and B cells, enter a node. Unmyelinated nerves enter the node at the hilus and run with blood vessels.

Other Lymphatic Tissue

In addition to such discretely organized tissue as lymph nodes and spleen, lymphatic tissue is associated with other tissues throughout the body. The wall of the alimentary tract is infiltrated with lymphatic tissue, evocative of the fact that developmentally this was the site where hematopoiesis first evolved. Lymphatic tissue, such as Peyer's patches, in the small intestine and the tonsils is well demarcated, whereas elsewhere it may diffusely infiltrate lamina propria and other layers. In addition to standard sites, lymphocytes, being migratory cells, may enter virtually any place in the body and with appropriate stimulation set up lymphatic loci.

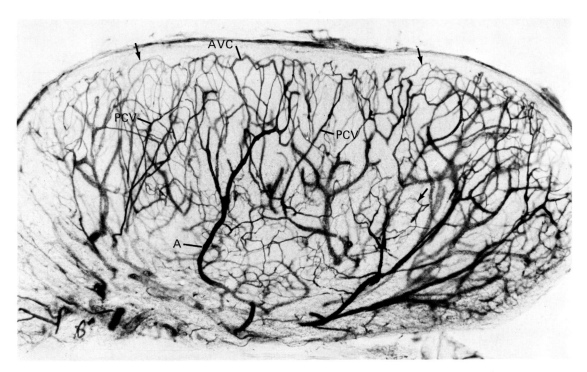

15–12 Lymph node of rat. This axillary lymph node has been perfused arterially by alcian blue and then sectioned and cleared to reveal the vasculature. Arteries **(A)** exhibit dense staining. Arteriovenous communications **(AVC)**, cortical and medullary capillaries **(arrows)**, and the high endothelial post capillary venules **(PCV)** are shown in the preparation. × 47. (From Anderson, A. D., and Anderson, N. D. 1975. Am. J. Pathol. 80:387.)

15–13 Schema of lymph node.

Afferent lymphatic vessels, some showing valves, pierce the capsule, and efferent lymphatics leave the node at the hilus. The nodular cortex consists of spherical lymphatic nodules, some of which contain germinal centers. The diffuse cortex lies between the nodules and deep to them. Within the center of the node lie the linear medullary cords, converging on the hilus. A subcapsular sinus, into which the afferent lymphatic vessels empty, lies beneath the full expanse of capsule. Radial sinuses run from the subcapsular sinus toward the hilus. They run along trabeculae, and, in the medulla, between medullary cords. Arteries enter the node at the hilus and branch richly, penetrating the node. Postcapillary venules tend to lie in the diffuse cortex. Veins leave the node at the hilus.

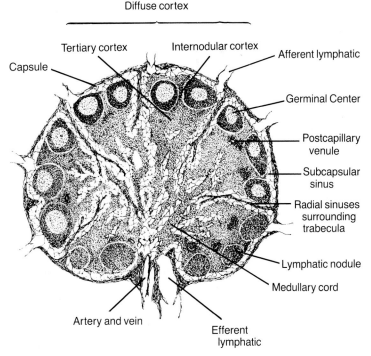

Diffuse cortex

Tertiary cortex

Internodular cortex

Capsule

Afferent lymphatic

Germinal Center

Postcapillary venule

Subcapsular sinus

Radial sinuses surrounding trabecula

Lymphatic nodule

Medullary cord

Artery and vein

Efferent lymphatic

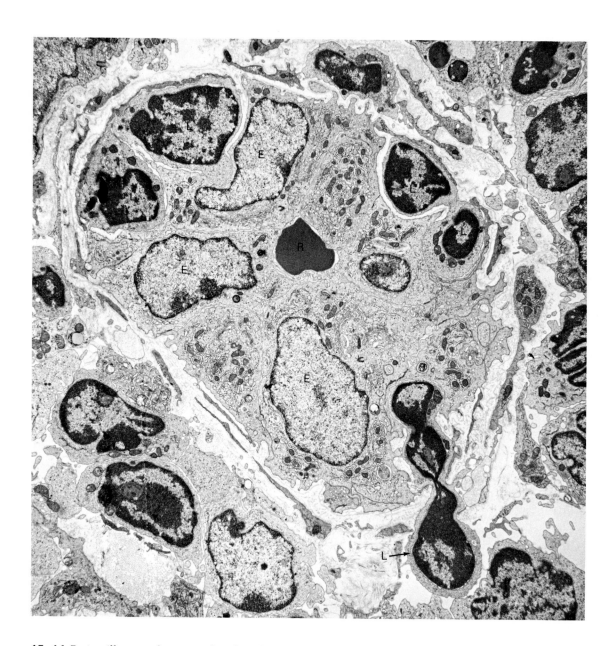

15–14 Postcapillary venules, mouse lymph node.
     The vessel has a high endothelium containing
lightly euchromatic nuclei **(E)**. The lumen is small
and contains an erythrocyte **(R).** The wall of the
venule is infiltrated by a number of lymphocytes
whose nuclei are heterochromatic and thus dense **(L).**
Note that one lymphocyte, its protoplasm beaded as a
result of being squeezed by the endothelium, appears
emerging from the venule and entering the
perivascular lymphatic cortex **(L→).** × 1,200. (From
the work of G. D. Levine.)

Development and Decline of Lymph Nodes

Lymph nodes appear in the human embryo during the third month along the course of lymphatic vessels. Lymphatic vessels at sites of
lymph node development become plexiform
(lymphatic sacs) and lymphocytes aggregate
around these sacs. Lymph nodes are not fully developed until several weeks postpartum, when
cortex and medulla differentiate and germinal
centers appear.
     Lymph nodes and spleen begin to atrophy at
the same time as thymus (Chap. 14), but the

15–15 A. Postcapillary venule, rat lymph node; scanning electron micrograph. Many lymphocytes lie on the endothelium, presumably about to penetrate between endothelial cells and through the wall of the venule into the surrounding cortex. Preparatory to crossing the wall, the lymphocytes appear to develop microvilli. × 563. **B.** At higher magnification, a lymphocyte is seen lying on the endothelium. The lymphocyte's microvilli appear to probe the endothelial surface. × 1,760. (From the work of A. O. Anderson and N. D. Anderson.)

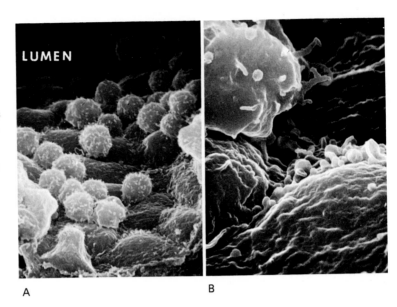

A   B

changes are quite gradual and subtle. In humans most nodes go on for 60 years or more with only slight atrophy, and they retain the capacity to enlarge throughout life.

15–16 Postcapillary venule in a mesenteric lymph node 15 min after the initiation of a transfusion. Labeled cells have penetrated the endothelium of the vessel but have not yet migrated into the node. **L,** lumen of the vessel. Exposure, 28 days. Methyl green–pyronin stain. × 1,200. (From Gowans, J. L., and Knight, E. J. 1964. Proc. R. Soc. Lond. [Biol.] 159:257.)

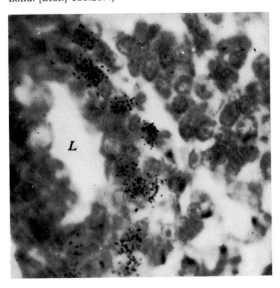

Functions of Lymph Nodes

Filtration and Phagocytosis. Lymph nodes constitute extensive filtration beds. The reticular meshwork, crisscrossing the sinuses and the parenchyma, acts as a mechanical filter. Flow in the lymphatic sinuses of lymph nodes is quite slow

15–17 Autoradiograph of thoracic duct cells that had been incubated in vitro with tritiated adenosine for 1 h at 37°C. Exposure, 14 days. Leishman stain. × 2,250. (From Gowans, J. L., and Knight, E. J. 1964. Proc. R. Soc. Lond. [Biol.] 159:257.)

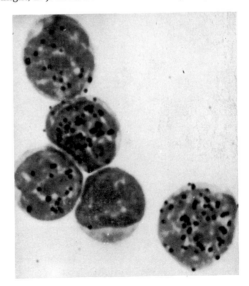

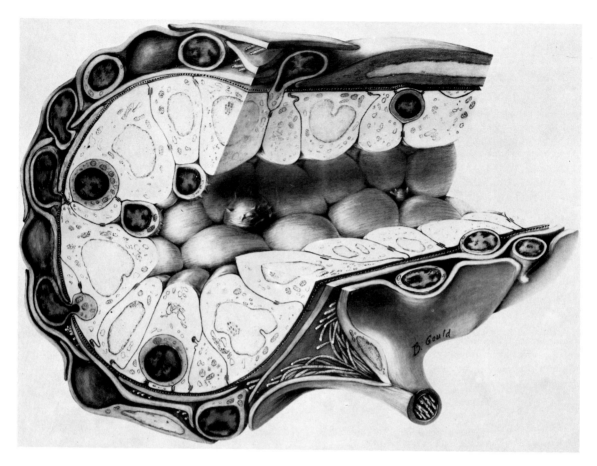

15–18 Postcapillary lymph node, artist's reconstruction. The high endothelium and the infiltration of the wall by lymphocytes are shown. (From the work of A. O. Anderson and N. D. Anderson.)

with many eddies, which favors phagocytosis. Fluid readily escapes the sinuses, moreover, and percolates through the parenchyma. Macrophages lie in the sinuses and in the parenchyma, and they can rapidly multiply and become activated. As they phagocytize, macrophages increase in volume; their bulk further impedes flow and thus enhances phagocytosis. Lymph nodes produce antibody (see below) and other substances that help to immobilize and agglutinate or lyse bacteria, facilitating filtration and phagocytosis. Drinker et al. (1934) perfused 5 ml of a serum-broth culture containing 600 million colonies per ml of hemolytic streptococci through a lymph node and collected perfusate at the efferent lymphatic vessels. When the perfusate was cultured, it was found to contain 4.5 million colonies/ml. The filtration efficiency was,

therefore, 99%. The efficiency of filtration makes lymph nodes vulnerable. If they fail to destroy the infectious agents or malignant cells that they concentrate, nodes become new foci and facilitate the spread of disease throughout the body.

Recirculation of Lymphocytes. Small T and B lymphocytes are part of the recirculating lymphocyte pool, traveling repeatedly through blood and lymphatic vessels and through lymph node, spleen, and other lymphatic tissue. Recirculating cells may enter a node through its arterial vessels, pass through capillaries, and reach postcapillary venules. They then pass through the walls of these venules into the parenchyma of the node. If they are T cells, they move to the diffuse cortex. B cells move to lymphatic nodules (Fig. 15–19). The lymphocytes remain in their characteristic sites for several hours and, if they do not engage in antibody production, they migrate to the medulla and leave the node through efferent lymphatics. Recirculating lymphocytes may also enter a node through afferent lymphatics, especially if the node is central and receives

15–19 Lymph node, mouse. Distribution of T and B lymphocytes as revealed by fluorescence immunocytochemistry. The T and B cells are specially stained in these frozen sections by antibodies to the surface of T and B cells, respectively. The antibody is conjugated to a fluorescent marker, visible by fluorescence microscopy. In **A,** the lymphatic nodules in the cortex are largely unstained, whereas the deep or tertiary cortex is deeply stained, indicating that it is the site of concentration of T lymphocytes. Note that the postcapillary venule is stained. In **B,** the cells of the lymphatic nodules are deeply stained, indicating that B lymphocytes are concentrated there. Note that the postcapillary venule is also stained, as are some cells in the tertiary cortex. This staining pattern reflects B-cell traffic from the postcapillary venule toward the lymphatic nodule. (See Fig. 16–22 for distribution of T and B lymphocytes in the spleen.) (From Weissman, I. L. 1975. Transpl. Rev. 24:159.)

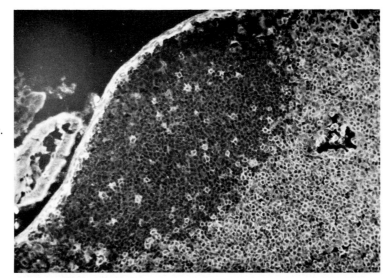

A

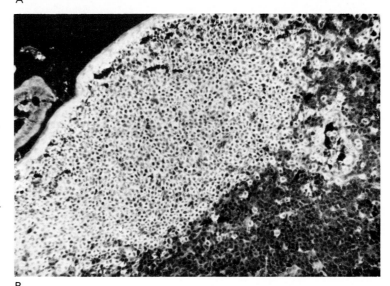

B

lymphocytes from more peripheral nodes. Transit time through a node in rodents is 4 to 6 h for T cells and somewhat longer for B cells. The recirculating lymphocytes enter veins through the thoracic ducts. They circulate in the blood stream until they eventually reach a lymph node (or other lymphatic tissue) and repeat the cycle. When T and B cells become engaged in antibody formation in a node, the pattern of recirculation is altered, as discussed below.

Immunological Functions. Lymph nodes produce antibody and engage in cellular immunity to regional antigen. Thus, antigen introduced into a footpad elicits an antibody response in a popliteal lymph node. This responsiveness of the lymph node to regional antigen complements that of the spleen, which responds to systemic (blood-borne) antigen. That lymphatic tissue produces antibody was shown by McMaster and Hudack in 1935, who injected antigen into the ears of rats and recovered antibody from the draining lymph nodes before it could be detected elsewhere. Two antigens were injected, one in each ear, and the antibody to each of the antigens was detected first in the isolateral node.

When antigen is first administered, a primary immune response follows that varies with the character of antigen, dose, and route of administration. With particulate antigens, such as bacteria or parts of bacteria, phagocytosis by macrophages is one of the earliest responses in a lymph node. The antigen is engulfed in the sinuses and in the medullary regions most conspicuously. However, antigen becomes concentrated rather rapidly around the primary nodules at the interface to T- and B-cell zones and then within the nodules. Soon the antigen disappears from other sites but remains in and around the lymphatic nodules, affixed to local macrophages and to antigen-presenting cells. Antigen thus held would seem able to interact with recirculating T and B cells as they move and sort themselves in the cortex of the node. This antigen processing enhances *clonal selection*, whereby the antigen *selects* T and B cells whose surface receptors "fit" with it. Selected T cells in the diffuse cortex and selected B cells in nodules proliferate to form *clones* by undergoing "blast transformation." These events occur within 24 h in a primary reaction.

Within several days, in a mounting reaction, antigen becomes more concentrated in the mantle zone and in germinal centers, held primarily by antigen-presenting cells. T cells undergoing blast transformation and proliferation in the diffuse cortex move into lymphatic nodules. There they interact both with B cells that have the appropriate receptors and with macrophages. These cell types proliferate and form a *germinal center*. As this happens, the small lymphocytes that have made up the primary nodule are forced to the periphery of the nodule and become the *mantle* or *crescent*. The resulting mantle and germinal center constitute a secondary nodule. By the fifth day of an active response, most of the activity may be in germinal centers. There, *effector B cells* undergoing transformation into plasma cells (the so-called *transitional cells*) produce considerable antibody and move toward the medullary cords as they complete their differentiation to plasma cells. Lymphocytes with immunological "memory" are produced (see below). Activated lymphocytes, both T and B, also release lymphokines, which have many actions. Lymphokines summon, detain, and activate macrophages and other cell types. They cause an increased vascular permeability, perhaps through intermediary mast cells and basophils, which leads to accumulation of perivascular fluid. The node is now tense and swollen. Over the next week or more the activity diminishes. Germinal centers remain for several weeks but show both an increasing proportion of macrophages that mop up and a decreasing proportion of activated lymphocytes. Plasma cells continue to accumulate in the medullary cords and live about 2 weeks, but their antibody output is low compared with that of transitional cells. In the process of antibody formation by effector B cells, there is increased production in the node of *memory B cells* (those which were not transformed to plasma cells) and of *memory T cells*. These cells join the recirculating pool of lymphocytes, augmenting the lymphocytes in the pool that had been initially responsive to the stimulating antigen.

On reexposure to antigen, a secondary reaction ensues. This time the lymph node reaction is more rapid, intense, and sustained, and the dominant feature is germinal center formation. As in the primary reaction, but after a longer period of time, the secondary reaction subsides: transitional cells synthesizing antibody in the germinal center die or are dispersed, macrophages increase in number and clean up, and the titer of antibody begins to fall. Macrophages within germinal centers contain a distinctive type of phagolysosome, called the *tingible* body, which includes nuclear material of phagocytized cells. When large numbers of macrophages containing tingible bodies are present in a germinal center they give an appearance that has been compared to a starry sky.

References and Selected Bibliography

General

Crabb E. D., and Kelsall, M. A. 1940. Organization of the mucosa and lymphatic structures in the rabbit appendix. J. Morphol. 67:351.

Fujita, T. 1978. Microarchitecture of reticular tissues. Reevaluation of the RES by scanning electron microscopy. Recent Adv. RES Res. 18:1.

Fujita, T., Miyoshi, M., and Murakami, T. 1972. Scanning electron microscope observation of the dog mesenteric lymph node. Z. Zellforsch. 133:147.

Porter, R., and Whelan J. (eds.). 191. Microenvironments in haemopoietic and lymphoid differentiation. CIBA Foundation Symposium 84.

Yoffey, J., and Courtice, F. 1956. Lymphatics, Lymph, and Lymphoid Tissue. Cambridge, Mass.: Harvard University Press.

Immune Response

Coons, A. H., Leduc, E. H., and Connolly, J. M. 1955. Studies on antibody production. I. A method for the histochemical demonstration of specific antibody and its application to a study of the hyperimmune rabbit. J. Exp. Med. 102:49.

Gastkemper, N. A., Wubbena, A. S., and Nieuwenhuis, P. 1979. Germinal centres and the B cell system: A search for the germinal centre precursor cell in the rat. *In* Adv. Biol. Med. 114:43. New York: Plenum Press.

Hanaoka, M. Nomoto, K., and Waksman, B. H., 1970. Appendix and IgM-antibody formation. I. Immune response and tolerance to bovine-Ig-globulin in irradiated, appendix-shielded rabbit. J. Immunol. 104:616.

Humphrey, J. H. 1976. The still unsolved germinal centre mystery. *In* Adv. Exp. Biol. Med. 66:711. New York: Plenum Press.

Klaus, G. G. B., Humphrey, J. H., Kinkl, A., and Dongworth, D. W., 1980. The follicular dendritic cell: Its role in antigen presentation in the generation of immunological memory. *In* Moller, G. (ed.), Imm. Rev. 53:3–28. Copenhagen: Munksgaard.

McMaster, P. D., and Hudack, S. 1935. The formation of agglutinins within lymph nodes. J. Exp. Med. 61:783.

Milstein, C. 1980. Monoclonal antibodies. Sci. Amer. 243:66.

Nieuwenhuis, P., and Lennert, K., 1980. Histophysiology of normal lymphoid tissue and immune reactions. *In* Van den Tweel et al. (eds.), Malignant Lymphoproliferative Diseases. The Hague: Martinus Nijhoff Publ., p. 3–12.

Ortega, L., and Mellors, R. 1957. Cellular sites of formation of gamma globulin. J. Exp. Med. 106:627.

Walesman, B. M., Ozer, M., and Blythman, M. 1973. Appendix and IgM antibody formation V. The functional anatomy of the rabbit appendix. Lab. Invest. 28:614.

Weissman, I. L. 1975. Development and distribution of immunoglobulin-bearing cells in mice. Transplant. Rev. 24:159.

Lymphocytes

Cho, Y., and De Bruyn, P. P. H. 1981. Transcellular migration of lymphocytes through the walls of the smooth surfaced squamous endothelial venules in the lymph node: Evidence for the direct entry of lymphocytes into the blood circulation of the lymph node. J. Ultrastruct. Res. 74:259.

De Sousa, M., Freitas, A., Huber, B., Cantor, H., and Boyse, E. A. 1979. Migratory patterns of the Ly subsets of T lymphocytes in the mouse. *In* Adv. Exp. Biol. Med. 114:51. New York: Plenum Press.

Gowans, J. L., and Knight, E. J. 1964. The route of recirculation of lymphocytes in the rat. Proc. R. Soc. Lond. (Biol) 159:257.

Gowans, J. L., McGregor, D., and Cowen, D. 1962. Initiation of immune responses by small lymphocytes. Nature (Lond). 196:651.

Nieuwenhuis, P. and Ford, W. L. 1976. Comparative migration of B- and T-lymphocytes in the rat spleen and lymph nodes. Cell. Immunol. 23:254.

Parrott, D. M. V., De Sousa, A. B., and East, J. 1966. Thymic dependent areas in the lymphoid organs of neonatally thymectomized mice. J. Exp. Med. 123:191.

Lymph Nodes

Clark, S. 1962. The reticulum of lymph nodes in mice studies with the electron microscope. Am. J. Anat. 110:217.

Drinker, C. K., Field, M. E., and Ward, H. K. 1934. The filtering capacity of lymph nodes. J. Exp. Med. 59:393.

Drinker, C. K., Wislocki, G. B., and Field, M. E. 1933. The structure of the sinuses in the lymph nodes. Anat. Rec. 56:261.

Han, S. 1961. The ultrastructure of the mesenteric lymph node of the rat. Am. J. Anat. 109:183.

Lymphatic Vessels

Crandall, L. A., Barker, S. B., and Graham, D. G. 1943. A study of the lymph flow from a patient with thoracic duct fistula. Gastroenterology 1:1040.

Forkert, P. G., Thliveris, J. A., and Bertalanffy, F. D. 1977. Structure of sinuses in the human lymph node. Cell Tissue Res. 183:115.

Leak, L. V., and Burke, J. F. 1968. Ultrastructural studies on the lymphatic anchoring filaments. J. Cell Biol. 36:129.

Vasculature

Anderson, A. O., and Anderson, N. D. 1975. Studies on the structure and permeability of the microvasculature in normal rat lymph nodes. Am. J. Pathol. 80:387.

Marchesi, V. T., and Gowans, J. L. 1964. The migration of lymphocytes through the endothelium of venules in lymph nodes: An electron microscope study. Proc. R. Soc. Lond. (Biol.) 159:283.

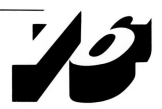

The Spleen

Leon Weiss

The spleen, weighing approximately 150 g in adult human beings, contains a specialized vasculature that modifies the circulating blood. There is no element of the blood, cellular or plasmal, that the spleen does not affect. It provides the proper hematopoietic microenvironment for the final differentiation of reticulocytes, platelets, T and B cells, and monocytes. It monitors the red blood cells of the circulation and destroys or modifies imperfect ones. It removes damaged or aged blood cells of all types. It sequesters monocytes from the blood, facilitates their transformation into macrophages, and holds them; they then impart enormous phagocytic capacity and other macrophage functions to the spleen. It receives T and B cells of the recirculating pool from the blood and sorts them into compartments, enabling them to interact with macrophages and antigen and to participate in immune responses. It stores as many as a third of the platelets of the body in a ready reserve. In certain species, it can also function as a reservoir for erythrocytes and granulocytes, delivering them rapidly to the blood when needed. The adult spleen is not essential to life, although its loss makes one more vulnerable to overwhelming infection. In some pathological conditions it may, in fact, eliminate or sequester circulating blood cells with such avidity that it must be removed to save life.

Structure of the Spleen

Capsule and Trabeculae

The human spleen is enclosed by a capsule of dense white connective tissue, a few millimeters in thickness. From the internal capsular surface a rich branching network of trabeculae subdivides the organ into communicating compartments several millimeters in each dimension (Fig. 16–1). The capsule contains relatively little muscle and is therefore incapable of the profound contraction that the muscular capsule of the spleen in dogs and cats exhibits. The capsule is indented medially at the hilus, where it is penetrated by blood vessels, lymphatic vessels, and nerves. Arterial vessels branch into the trabeculae and from there into the pulp or parenchyma of the organ. Veins and lymphatics also travel in the trabeculae, entering from the pulp and running out.

Splenic Pulp

The tissue enclosed within the capsule and trabeculae is the splenic pulp (Figs. 16–2 to 16–4). Much of it is red, owing to the presence of erythrocytes, and it is called red pulp. There are two types of spleen, those that contain vascular sinuses and those that do not. In sinusal spleens, of which the human spleen is an example, red pulp is made up of four vascular structures: slender nonanastomosing arterial vessels; large, branching thin-walled venous vessels called venous sinuses (or sinusoids); and thin plates or partitions of cellular tissue lying between the sinuses, called splenic cords. The venous sinuses flow into pulp veins. In nonsinusal spleens, like that of the cat, venous sinuses are absent. Blood flows through arterial vessels, pulp spaces, and veins.

Grossly visible zones of tightly packed lymphocytes also occur in the pulp and constitute the white pulp of the spleen. White pulp assumes two formations. One is cylindrical and surrounds major arterial branches of the splenic pulp as periarterial lymphatic sheaths. The other form is nodular and comprises the lymphatic nodules, which lie within the periarterial lymphatic sheaths (Fig. 16–4). Immune responses in the spleen are initiated in the white pulp. The splenic pulp at the junction of white pulp and red pulp is called the marginal zone. It is the site of high blood traffic where the distinctive blood cell processing of the spleen is begun.

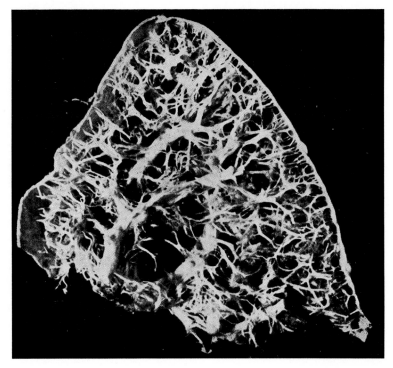

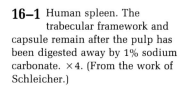

16–1 Human spleen. The trabecular framework and capsule remain after the pulp has been digested away by 1% sodium carbonate. ×4. (From the work of Schleicher.)

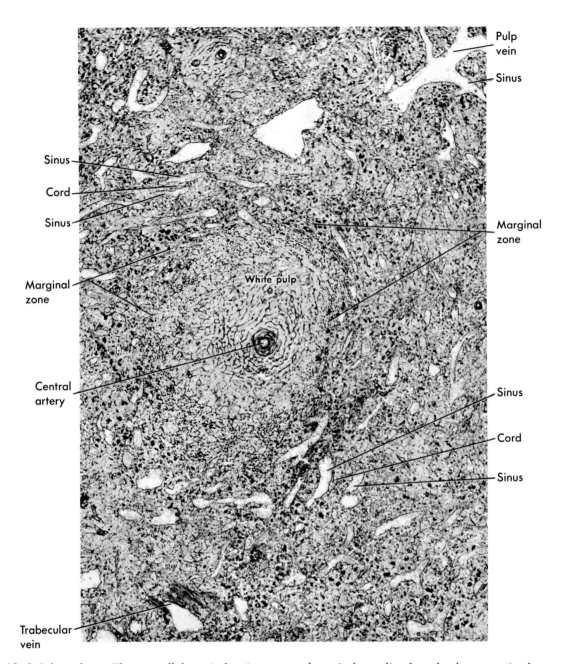

Labels on image: Pulp vein, Sinus, Sinus, Cord, Sinus, Marginal zone, Marginal zone, White pulp, Central artery, Sinus, Cord, Sinus, Trabecular vein

16–2 Spleen of a rat. The extracellular reticulum is stained by the PAS reaction. The white pulp contains a darkly outlined central artery. Note the circumferential pattern of the reticulum of white pulp. A marginal zone surrounds the white pulp and contains a relatively dense meshwork of reticulum and many darkly stained cells. Beyond the white pulp and marginal zone lies the red pulp, accounting for most of the splenic volume. The clear spaces represent splenic sinuses, for the most part, but also pulp veins and trabecular veins. The splenic cords constitute the relatively solid tissue lying between the sinuses. × 225. (From Weiss, L. 1959. J. Anat. 93:465.)

16-3 Spleen of a hedgehog. In this low-power field, the white pulp, red pulp, blood outflow tract, and splenic mesentery are shown. The white pulp, occupying a relatively small volume, surrounds a central artery. The red pulp occupies most of the field. It is made up almost entirely of relatively clear spaces, the splenic sinuses, which form an anastomosing system of venous vessels. The splenic cords, darkly stained tissue lying between the sinuses, consist of a reticular meshwork that contains blood cells and macrophages and receives arterial terminations. Blood is carried out of the spleen through trabecular veins, which drain into the splenic vein. Splenic veins leave the spleen at the hilus and enter the splenic mesentery. At the **arrow,** splenic sinuses empty into a pulp vein that drains into a trabecular vein. The marginal zone lies between white pulp and red pulp. The mesentery contains a branch of the splenic artery that will enter the spleen at the hilus. × 150. (From Janout, V., and Weiss, L. 1972. Anat. Rec. 172:197.)

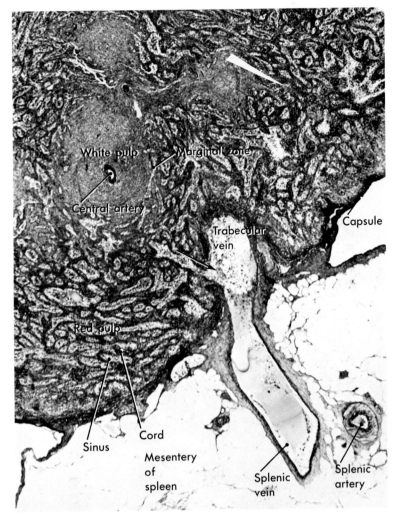

Blood Flow

Blood enters the spleen by way of splenic arteries that pass through the hilus. A splenic artery branches into trabeculae as *trabecular arteries,* which turn out of the trabeculae and enter the pulp. In the pulp, they are surrounded by *periarterial lymphatic sheaths.* As an artery travels through the periarterial lymphatic sheath as the *central artery,* it sends out many branches; some supply the lymphatic nodules within the sheath. In the human spleen, most branches travel to the periphery of the sheath and terminate in the marginal zone. The central artery itself runs out into the red pulp and terminates in cords. In the red pulp and in the marginal zone, blood flows through cords and enters splenic sinuses, which are tributaries of veins of the pulp. These veins

enter trabeculae as trabecular veins. At the hilus, the trabecular veins are continuous with splenic veins, which drain the organ. The circulation of the spleen has been difficult to analyze and it will be discussed more fully below, after the structure of the pulp is described.

Lymphatic vessels lie in white pulp, girdling the central artery (Figs. 16–4 and 16–5). Lymphatics run into trabeculae and out of the spleen to drain into lymph nodes in the splenic mesentery.

White Pulp

The white pulp of the spleen is a lymphatic tissue analogous to the cortex of lymph nodes. It consists of lymphocytes, macrophages, and other free cells lying in a specialized reticular mesh-

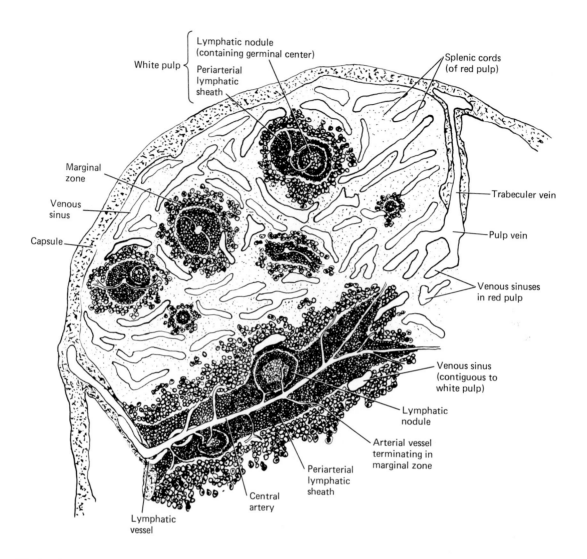

Lymphatic nodule
(containing germinal center)

White pulp

Periarterial
lymphatic
sheath

Splenic cords
(of red pulp)

Marginal
zone

Venous
sinus

Capsule

Trabeculer vein

Pulp vein

Venous sinuses
in red pulp

Venous sinus
(contiguous to
white pulp)

Lymphatic
nodule

Arterial vessel
terminating in
marginal zone

Periarterial
lymphatic
sheath

Central
artery

Lymphatic
vessel

16–4 Schematic view of the organization of the human spleen. The white pulp has two components: periarterial lymphatic sheaths and lymphatic nodules. The latter may be made up of a germinal center and a surrounding mantle zone. The white pulp is surrounded by the marginal zone. The remainder of the tissue depicted is the red pulp, which consists primarily of splenic sinuses separated by splenic cords. The pattern of blood flow is as follows. A trabecular artery enters the white pulp and becomes the central artery. The central artery passes through white pulp and gives rise to many branches. A few end within white pulp; some supply the germinal center and mantle zone of the secondary nodule. Most terminate at the periphery of the white pulp, emptying in or near the marginal zone. A number of arterial vessels emerge from the white pulp, pass into the marginal zone, reach the red pulp, and curve back to empty into the marginal zone. Some arterial branches, in addition to the main stem of the central artery, run into the red pulp. Almost all terminate in the cords. Here, too, variation exists. Some arterial vessels terminate in a cord close against a sinus wall, whereas others terminate in the midst of a cord, away from any sinus. Arterial vessels may terminate as capillaries or as somewhat larger vessels. Some arterial vessels may bear sheaths shortly before termination. The sinuses drain into pulp veins, which, in turn, drain into trabecular veins. A sinus may abut the white pulp and receive lymphocytes or other free cells that migrate from white pulp across its wall and into its lumen. Efferent lymphatic vessels lie about the proximal portion of the central artery and run out of the spleen through the trabeculae. (From Weiss, L., and Tavossoli, M. 1970. Semin. Hematol. 7:372.)

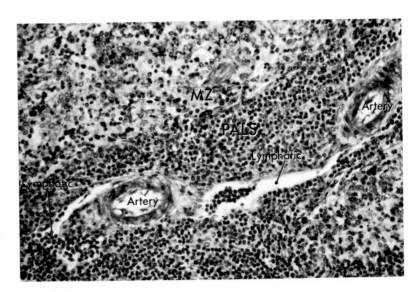

16–5 Spleen of a hedgehog. Lymphatic vessels are shown in this field. They lie within the periarterial lymphatic sheath **(PALS)** of white pulp in relation to the central artery, two branches of which are shown. The PALS consists of a reticular meshwork obscured by many lymphocytes crowded together. Outside the PALS is the marginal zone **(MZ).** ×950. (From Janout, V., and Weiss, L. 1972. Anat. Rec. 172:197.)

work. The periarterial lymphatic sheaths are cylinders that axially surround the central artery. Their reticular meshwork tends to be arranged in circumferential layers around the central artery, with a more prominent circumferential reticulum at their periphery (Figs. 16–6, 16–9, and 16–10). Lymphocytes are the most numerous of the free cells packed in these sheaths. They are predominantly T cells of the recirculating pool.

Periarterial lymphatic sheaths persist around arterial vessels, tapering down as the vessels branch and become finer. The sheaths are quite attenuated when the arterial vessels they surround become small arterioles. Lymphatic nodules are spherical or ovoid, resembling nodules of the cortex of lymph nodes. They lie within the periarterial lymphatic sheath, often at arterial branchings. B cells are concentrated in nodules.

16–6 A sketch of the meshwork of white pulp. Lymphocytes and other free cells are not included. The reticular cells are indicated as nucleated outlines. The reticular fibers, such as are stained in Fig. 16–2, are stippled. Virtually the entire field is taken by a cross section of the periarterial lymphatic sheath (PALS), in the center of which is the cross section of the central artery. Near the central artery the reticular meshwork may not be markedly specialized, while at the periphery it is circumferential (see Figs. 16–2 and 16–9). To the left of the central artery, the reticular meshwork supports a small lymphatic nodule supplied by several arterioles. A large branch of the central artery curves down and to the right, reaching the red pulp where it bifurcates **(1).** (See Fig. 16–11.) Another large branch travels toward 12 o'clock and ends in the marginal zone as a sheathed capillary **(2).** Another vessel arches toward 2 o'clock and opens into the marginal zone **(3).** (From Weiss, L. 1972. Cells and Tissues of the Immune System. Englewood Cliffs, N.J.: Prentice-Hall, Inc.)

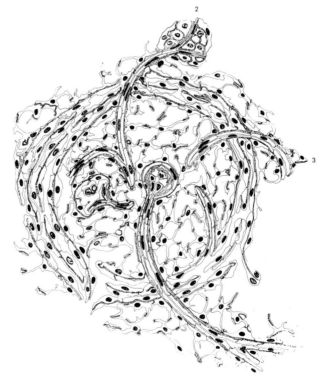

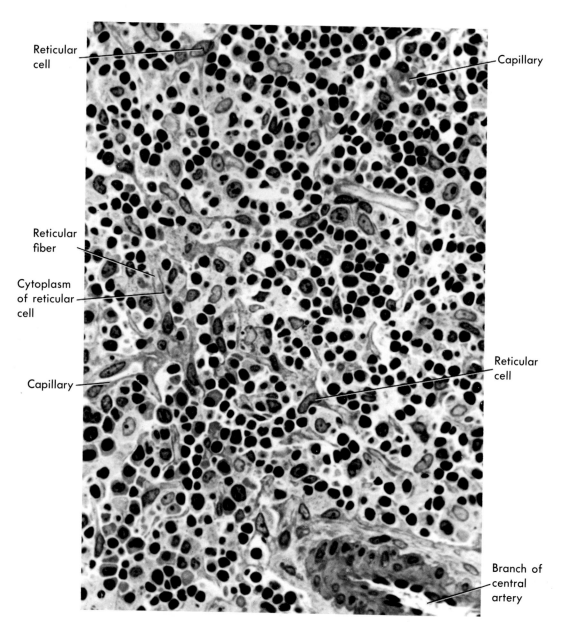

Reticular cell

Capillary

Reticular fiber

Cytoplasm of reticular cell

Reticular cell

Capillary

Branch of central artery

16–7 Spleen of a rabbit, periarterial lymphatic sheath of white pulp. A large branch of the central artery lies in the right lower corner. The larger part of the field consists of a reticular meshwork within which lies the small, densely stained round lymphocytes and related free cells. The meshwork is made of branching reticular cells and reticular fibers. The reticular cells ensheath the more lightly stained reticular fibers. Small blood vessels are present in places in this field. Their adventitial layers are continuous with the reticular meshwork, as are the adventitial layers of the branch of the central artery in the right lower corner. × 600. (From Weiss, L. 1964. Bull. Johns Hopkins Hosp. 115:99.)

Splenic nodules, like those of lymph nodes, may become secondary nodules by developing germinal centers. Antigen-presenting cells (page 535) are present in the white pulp. Lymphatic nodules cause periarterial lymphatic sheaths to bulge unevenly and thus force the central artery to assume an eccentric position.

Vascular Supply of White Pulp

The central artery is a medium-sized muscular artery that gives off branches as it runs through the periarterial lymphatic sheath (Figs. 16–3,

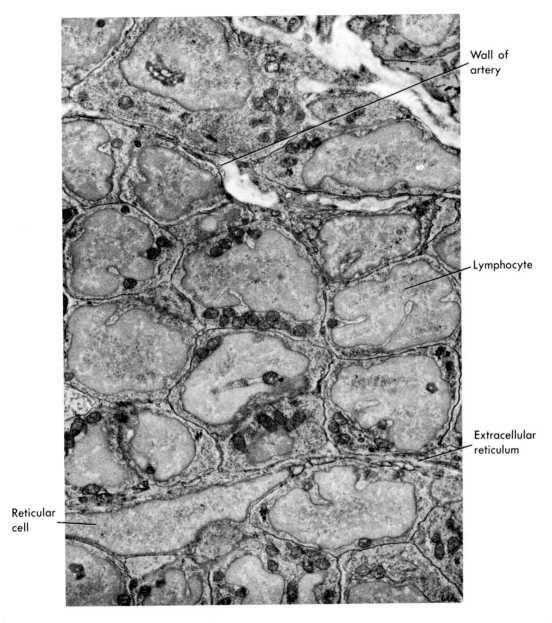

Wall of
artery

Lymphocyte

Extracellular
reticulum

Reticular
cell

16–4, 16–6, and 16–7 to 16–9). The branches tend to run radially toward the periphery of the white pulp. Many go beyond the white pulp and empty into the marginal zone. Some travel farther, reach red pulp, and terminate there. Lymphatic nodules are supplied by a deep and superficial set of branches from the central artery. Snook has described a distinctive arrangement in human spleen wherein lymphatic nodules are supplied by recurrent arteries curving back from red pulp. Efferent lymphatic vessels originate deep in white pulp. They converge on the central artery and its branches and wind around them,

16–8 Spleen of a rat, periarterial lymphatic sheath of white pulp. This electron micrograph illustrates the relationships of an arterial vessel, lymphocytes, and the reticular meshwork. The adventitia of a large branch of the central artery is in the upper part of the field. Small lymphocytes are present, tightly packed together. Note that their scanty cytoplasm is rich in ribonucleoprotein and in mitochondria but lacks endoplasmic reticulum. These cells are preponderantly T lymphocytes (see Fig. 16–22). A reticular cell in the lower part of the field is associated with a small segment of extracellular reticulum. × 15,000. (From Weiss, L. 1964. Bull. Johns Hopkins Hosp. 115:99.)

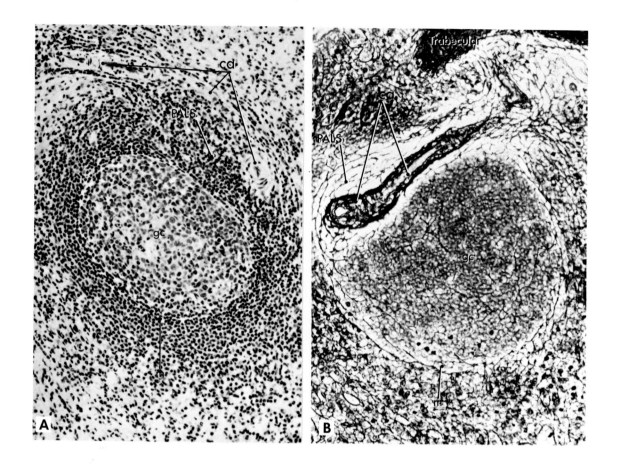

16–9 Human spleen, white pulp. **A.** Where the cells are stained with Giemsa stain, a central artery **(ca)** surrounded by the small lymphocyte-rich periarterial lymphatic sheath **(PALS)** curves into the field from the left. At the left leader it is cut in longitudinal section; at the right leader, in cross section. Hanging from the lower border of the PALS is a large lymphatic nodule, consisting of a large germinal center surrounded by a dense mantle **(m)** of small lymphocytes. **B.** In a reticulum preparation, in which the extracellular reticulum is blackened by silver, a similar field is shown. A central artery **(ca)** curves in from the right. It probably comes from the nearby trabecula. The central artery is surrounded by a PALS. Note the circumferential pattern of the reticulum of the PALS around the central artery. Again, a large lymphatic nodule hangs from the PALS. The periphery of the nodule, constituting the mantle **(m)** of small lymphocytes, actually represents the PALS, which has been carried out by the presence of the large germinal center **(gc)**. × 450. (From the preparation of K. Richardson.)

moving toward the trabeculae with their contents flowing into trabecular lymphatics. These lymphatic vessels are tributaries of larger collecting vessels that leave the spleen and empty into lymph nodes in the splenic mesentery and near the celiac plexus.

Marginal Zone

The marginal zone, lying between white pulp and red pulp, is bound centrally (on its white pulp aspect) by the outermost circumferential lamella of the white pulp. On its periphery or red pulp aspect it blends into the cords of red pulp. The reticular meshwork of the marginal zone is quite fine in human spleen. Many arterial vessels open into the marginal zone. They may terminate in a funnel-shaped orifice and often bifurcate just before ending. Venous sinuses regularly come near or into the marginal zone. The marginal zone is a site of heavy blood traffic and filtration, and much of the splenic processing of blood begins there.

Red Pulp

Red pulp in human spleen is a reticular mesh-work supplied by arteries and drained by venous sinuses (Figs. 16–3, 16–4, and 16–10 to 16–19). The venous sinuses form an anastomosing sys-tem in the meshwork. As a result, the reticular meshwork takes the form of a branching system of cords lying between the sinuses. After it dis-tributes branches to the white pulp and marginal zone, the attenuated main stem of the central ar-tery runs on into the cords of red pulp and branches into straight nonanastomosing slender vessels, about 25 μm in outside diameter, called *penicilli.* Arterial vessels open into the reticular meshwork of the cords. They do not open into the venous sinuses.

Shortly before they terminate, arterial capil-laries may be modified by running through a sheath of macrophages supported in a reticular meshwork. (Figs. 16–20 and 16–21). The most commonly used term for these sheaths has been *ellipsoid* because the sheaths may have that shape, but they are often spherical, cylindrical, or irregular. Blue and Weiss have suggested the term *periarterial macrophage sheath* because it is anatomically and functionally descriptive and it is consistent with the useful term *periarterial lymphatic sheath,* which describes an analogous structure. Sheaths may be spongy because cells are loosened by plasma infiltration, or they may be tightly compressed. Erythrocytes, granulo-cytes, and other blood cells may be present in the sheath. The periarterial macrophage sheaths may represent a major population of macro-phages in the spleen. Well-developed sheaths possess extraordinary phagocytic capacity and are major sites of clearance of blood-borne parti-cles in the red pulp. They may, moreover, play a role in controlling blood flow in the spleen. Sheaths vary in development depending on the species. In the dog and cat they are very promi-nent. In rabbits they are absent. Periarterial mac-rophage sheaths in the human spleen are rela-tively small, and not every arterial capillary bears one. In spleens that lack periarterial mac-rophage sheaths, clearance functions are handled by macrophages in the marginal zone and red pulp. In some species, such as the horse, sheaths contain antigen-presenting cells.

Splenic cords, as indicated, are part of the vascular pathway, receiving blood from arterial vessels and conveying it to venous sinuses. The vascular pathway through the cords may be long,

where arterial vessels terminate some distance from the vascular sinus, or it may be short, where arterial vessels terminate close to the wall of vascular sinuses. Functions other than blood flow may occur in splenic cords. Erythropoiesis and, to a lesser degree, granulocytopoiesis may occur there. This hematopoiesis is not unusual in rodents but happens only pathologically in human spleen. Destruction of blood cells, in par-ticular, old or damaged erythrocytes, also occurs in splenic cords and may be evident by the pres-ence of erythrophagocytic macrophages.

16–10 Spleen of a rat. The periphery of white pulp (the periarterial lymphatic sheath, PALS) is present. On the left are the closely packed cells of the PALS. A large macrophage may be seen. Its location at the periphery of white pulp is characteristic. The PALS has a well-defined rim of concentric strands of reticulum, running from top to bottom of this field (between **arrows**). This rim is well shown in silver preparations in which the extracellular reticulum is stained (see Fig. 16–9). The marginal zone is on the right. × 19,000. (From Weiss, L. 1964. Bull. Johns Hopkins Hosp. 115:99.)

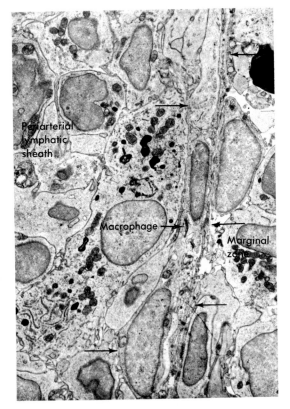

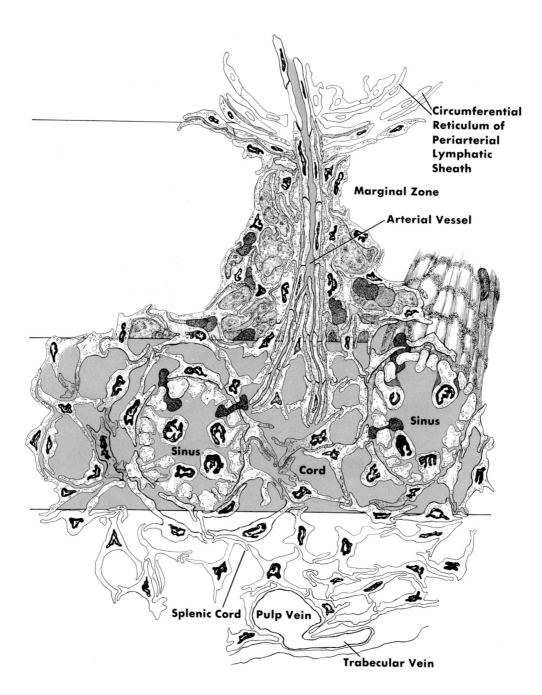

Circumferential Reticulum of Periarterial Lymphatic Sheath

Marginal Zone

Arterial Vessel

Sinus

Sinus

Cord

Splenic Cord   **Pulp Vein**

Trabecular Vein

16–11 Spleen. Schematic view of artery leaving the periarterial lymphatic sheath white pulp and entering red pulp. It enters a splenic cord and bifurcates between two sinuses. (From Weiss, L. 1972. The Cells and Tissues of the Immune System. Englewood Cliffs, N.J.: Prentice-Hall, Inc.)

Splenic Sinuses

Splenic sinuses (Figs. 16–2 to 16–4 and 16–11 to 16–19) are long, anastomosing vascular channels, 35 to 40 μm in diameter, with a unique endothelium and basement membrane. The endothelial cells are elongate with tapered ends and lie parallel to the long axis of the sinus. In cross section through sinuses, therefore, the endothe-

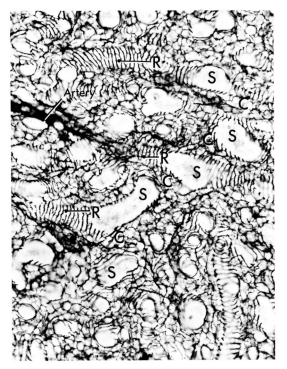

16–12 Red pulp of human spleen, reticulum stain.
△   Sinuses are present as clear spaces **(S).** Their basement membrane is exposed as consisting primarily of "ring fibers" **(R)**, deeply stained. This membrane is continuous with the reticular fibers of the cords **(C).** An artery entering from the left appears to open into the cord. × 600. (From the preparation of K. Richardson.)

lial cells are cut in cross section. They lie side by side and are separated by a slitlike space. Tight junctional complexes occur regularly along their lateral surfaces. Endothelial cells contain bundles of microfilaments that run longitudinally in the basal cytoplasm. Intermediate (100 Å) filaments are distributed basally and throughout the cytoplasm. The luminal surface of endothelium is rich in micropinocytotic vesicles. Blood cells flowing through the red pulp cross the wall of splenic sinuses between endothelial cells.

The endothelium lies on a basement membrane, which may be deeply stained in the periodic acid Schiff reaction or impregnated by silver. The basement membrane is perforated by large, regularly arranged uniform polygonal apertures or fenestrae so that what little material remains of the basement membrane is reduced to slender strands that separate and outline the ap-

16–13 Rabbit spleen, red pulp. Sections of two
▽   sinuses with intervening cords are present in this light micrograph. The basement membrane, stained deeply with the PAS reaction, is interrupted (see Figs. 16–11, 16–12, and 16–19) in this section because of its fenestrated character. The cords are crowded with macrophages. Reticular cells and PAS-stained reticular fibers are present in the cords. An arterial vessel that opens into a cord is also present. PAS-hematoxylin stain. × 1,200. (From Weiss, L. 1959. J. Anat. 93:465.)

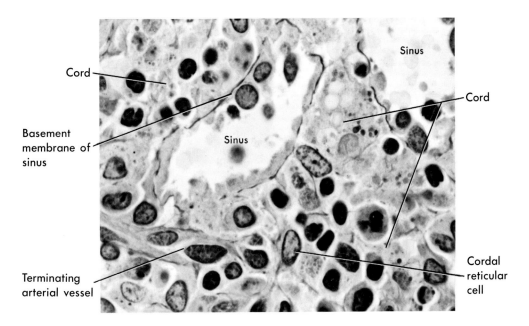

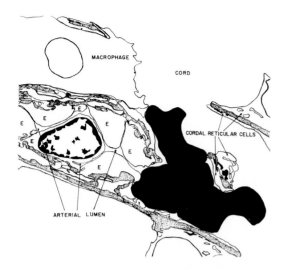

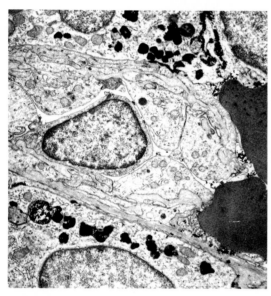

16–14 Spleen of a rabbit, red pulp. An arterial vessel ends in a cord. This vessel is typical of many terminating arterial vessels in red pulp. It is a small arteriole. Its endothelium (**E** in tracing) is high. Its lumen and the surrounding red pulp contain Thorotrast, which was injected intravenously several minutes before splenectomy. About two layers of extracellular reticulum (**stippled** in tracing) are present in the vessel wall. The inner one underlies the endothelium and constitutes a basement membrane. Portions of two macrophages lie above and below the vessel. The vessel opens to the right, and several erythrocytes lie just outside the orifice. × 18,000. (From Weiss, L. 1963. Am. J. Anat. 113:51.)

ertures (Figs. 16–11, 16–12, and 16–19). In a surface view, the basement membrane looks like a net. In human basement membrane, the transverse component is heavy and the longitudinal links relatively slight. The arrangement can be likened to a barrel in which the wooden staves correspond to the endothelium and the hoops to the basement membrane. With the electron microscope, the basement membrane is seen to consist of an extracellular granular material that may contain a few collagenous fibers. Its composition thus resembles that of reticular fibers and, indeed, reticular fibers of the cords surrounding splenic sinuses are continuous with the basement membrane of the sinuses (Figs. 16–11, 16–15, and 16–19). Reticular cells lie over the outside surface of the basement membrane of vascular sinuses, occupying an adventitial position. These reticular cells extend branches into the surrounding cords and are thereby part of the cordal reticular meshwork. They are associated with, and probably produce, reticular fibers.

The interendothelial slits of vascular sinuses constitute a major component in the vascular pathway through the red pulp. Blood passes out of arterial endings through the cords and through these interendothelial slits. From here it goes into the lumen of the vascular sinuses and then into splenic veins. In spleens without vascular sinuses, such as the cat's, blood flows from arterial terminations through the reticular meshwork of pulp spaces, a tissue comparable to splenic cords, and then is taken up by pulp veins.

Splenic Veins

Sinuses are tributaries of pulp veins. The transition of sinus into vein can be quite abrupt, the latter having a flat endothelium and a basement membrane without apertures. Blood cells do not cross the wall of pulp veins. These veins flow into trabecular veins that drain into the splenic veins, which leave the organ destined for the portal vein. Splenic vein blood may be rich in macrophages, which are undoubtedly filtered from the circulation by the liver and, should they pass the liver, by the lungs.

Embryology

The spleen originates in the dorsal mesogastrium at about 5-mm crown–rump length (CRL) in human embryos. At 40-mm CRL the spleen consists of an encapsulated cellular meshwork. By 55-

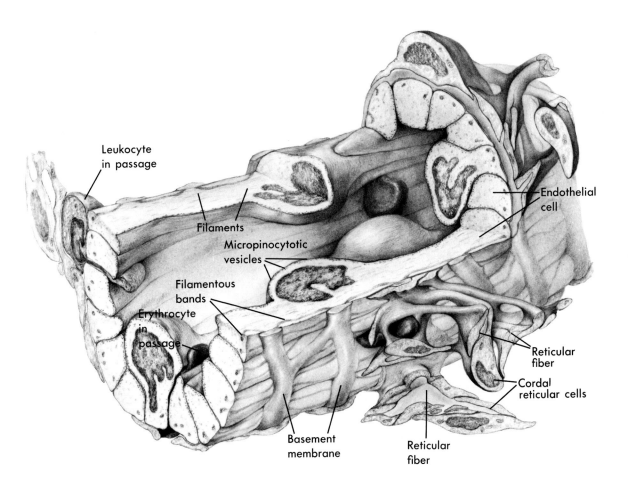

Leukocyte
in passage

Filaments

Micropinocytotic
vesicles

Filamentous
bands

Erythrocyte
in
passage

Endothelial
cell

Reticular
fiber

Cordal
reticular cells

Basement
membrane

Reticular
fiber

16–15 A schematic drawing of a human splenic sinus in red pulp. The endothelial cells are tapered rods that lie side by side with their long axis parallel to the long axis of the vessel. Virtually all arterial vessels end in the surrounding cords without direct connection to the sinuses. Accordingly, blood entering the vascular sinus must enter from the surrounding cord, squeezing through the slitlike spaces between sinus endothelial cells. Note that several blood cells in passage across the sinus wall are shown. The endothelial cells show several distinctive cytological features. These features include a row of pinocytotic vesicles just beneath the plasma membrane on the luminal and lateral surfaces, and two sets of cytoplasmic filaments. One set of filaments, rather loosely organized, runs longitudinally through the cytoplasm. The other set is tightly organized into dense bands in the basal cytoplasm. These bands arch between strands of the basement membrane. They appear to insert into the plasma membrane where it overlies the basement membrane and then continue through the plasma membrane into the substance of the basement membrane. These filaments are probably part of the cytoskeletal system, which stiffens the basal cytoplasm and maintains the shape of endothelial cells and the slitlike interendothelial space. They, or the other set of filaments, may be contractile. They play an important role in the spleen's capacity to recognize damaged blood cells and destroy or modify them (see text).

The basement membrane is fenestrated, having heavy strandlike transverse "ring" components and lighter longitudinal strands joining the rings. The large fenestrae or apertures in the basement membrane leave ample unimpeded space for blood cells to pass through the sinus wall. The cordal surface of the basement membrane is covered by cordal reticular cells, which branch into the surrounding cord. (From Chen, L. T., and Weiss, L. 1972. Am. J. Anat. 134:425.)

558

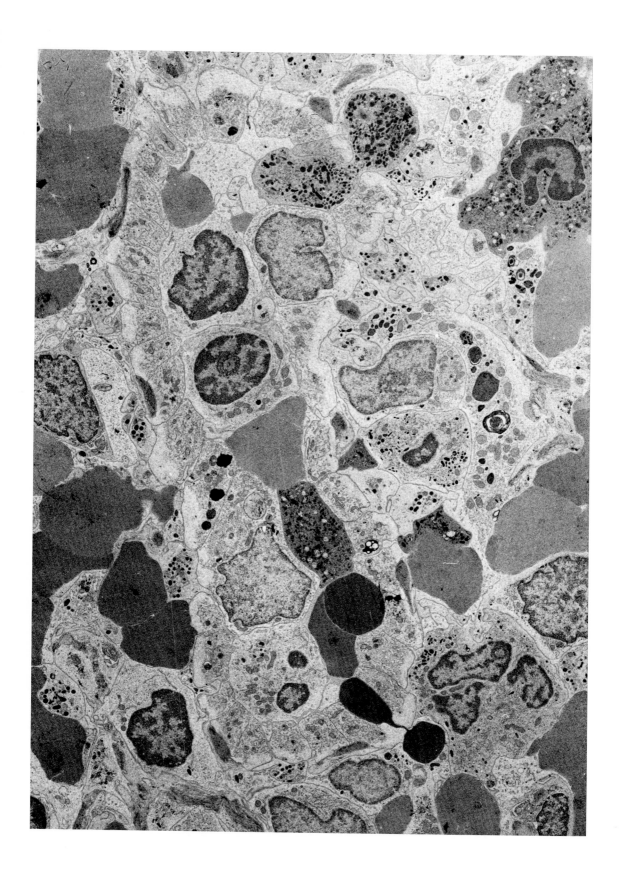

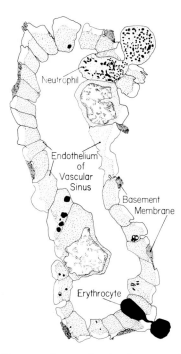

Neutrophil

Endothelium
of
Vascular
Sinus

Basement
Membrane

Erythrocyte

16–16 Human spleen, red pulp. A venous sinus occupies most of this field, but does not stand out because it is collapsed. Its wall is being crossed by an erythrocyte and neutrophil. Use above reduced tracing as key. Courtesy of Robert M. Powell

mm CRL, vascular sinuses are present and the meshwork is much looser, containing many free blood cells and macrophages. A rich vascular supply quickly develops. By 100-mm CRL, reticular cells tend to lay out the plan of the spleen and assume a circumferential pattern around arteries, defining the periarterial lymphatic sheaths and marginal zones. Soon thereafter, lymphocytes move into the periarterial sheaths, which are rather clearly developed after the first half of gestation. In the first trimester, the human fetal spleen is erythropoietic and myelopoietic. These activities fade after the fifth prenatal month, preempted successively by the liver and marrow.

Functions of the Spleen

The Circulation of Blood Through the Spleen

In most tissues of the body, blood flows through tubular blood vessels, and one can intuitively correlate the anatomy of the vascular bed with the physiology of actual blood flow. However, in some vascular beds, as in the cavernous tissue of the secondary sex organs and especially in the red pulp of the spleen, the anatomy is highly distinctive and correlations of structure and function are difficult to make. In order to understand the circulation of the spleen it is necessary to distinguish the structure of the vascular bed, determined by anatomical methods, from the nature of blood flow, determined by physiological methods.

Students of the spleen have wrestled with a major question about the anatomy of the vascular bed of red pulp: is the circulation open or closed? That is, do the arterial vessels connect directly to venous vessels, with endothelial continuity (closed circulation)? Or do the arterial vessels terminate and empty into the cords or pulp spaces, with the blood flowing through these spaces and then through the walls of venous vessels (open circulation)? Alternatively, is the circulation through the red pulp partly open and partly closed?

The overwhelming evidence is that the vascular pathway through the red pulp of the spleen, whether of the sinusal or nonsinusal type, is anatomically open. The key evidence is as follows: Arterial terminations can be seen by light microscopy and electron microscopy to open into the cords or pulp spaces, and blood is found there. Blood cells, moreover, may be regularly observed crossing the wall of vascular sinuses through interendothelial slits. No one has convincingly demonstrated endothelial continuity in sectioned material between arterial capillaries and venous sinuses or pulp veins.

Nonetheless, a number of investigators have concluded that the circulation through the red pulp of the spleen is closed, or that some arterial vessels do empty into sinuses. Let us consider the evidence for these conclusions. Knisely, whose work in the 1930s had great impact, studied the circulation in living spleen by exteriorizing the organ, maintaining its circulation intact, transilluminating it, and cooling it through a hollow quartz rod. He concluded that the circulation was closed. Several groups confirmed his work; others did not. But study of the living spleen is not primarily a study of the anatomical arrangements because this approach lacks the resolution to define endothelium and other cell structures critically. It is, rather, a study of blood flow. For example, Knisely studied circulation through the kitten spleen. This spleen contains no vascular sinuses. Arterial terminations are

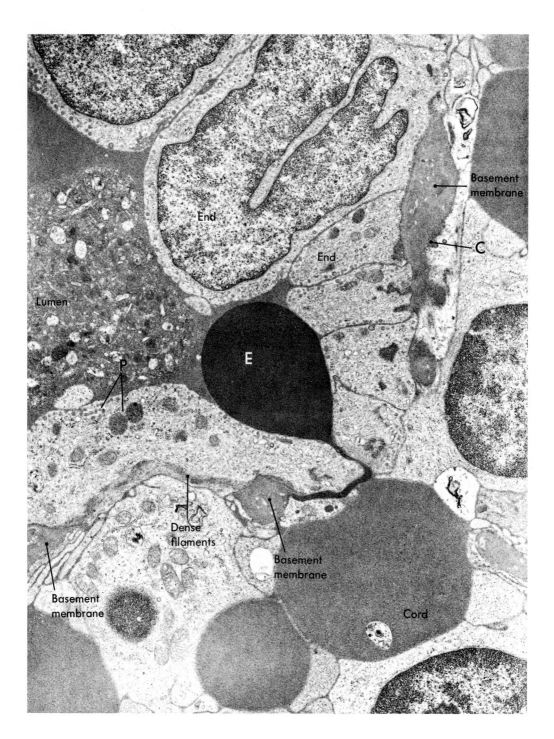

16–17 Human spleen, red pulp. An erythrocyte **(E)** passes from a cord and through the sinus wall between endothelial cells **(End)** into the lumen of the sinus. The erythrocyte is drawn into a thin strand as it passes through the mural slit. The endothelial cells contain many pinocytotic vesicles **(P)** at the luminal surface and dense filaments in the basal cytoplasm, which arches across the fenestrae of the basement membrane. Small portions of cordal reticular cells applied to the abluminal surface of the basement membrane are present. The cord is filled with erythrocytes and other free cells. × 10,000. (From Chen, L. T., and Weiss, L. 1972. Am. J. Anat. 134:425.)

16–18 Rat spleen, red pulp, showing the surface of the endothelium facing the lumen of a vascular sinus. The vessel runs from left to right, bifurcating on the right. The endothelial cells lie side by side, their long axis running from left to right. The cells bulge into the lumen in their nuclear zone. There appears to be no interendothelial space. At the curved **arrow** a red cell appears to be passing through the wall of the vascular sinus by squeezing between endothelial cells. Compare with Fig. 16–17 and see discussion in text. × 1,000. (From Weiss, L. 1974. Blood. 43:665.)

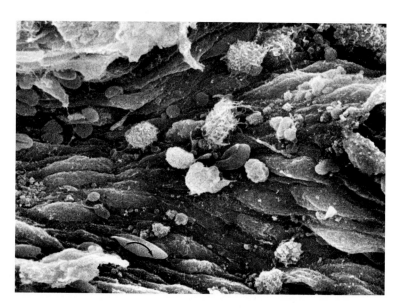

16–19 Human spleen. Reconstuction of extracellular reticulum of red pulp. Four sinuses are present in this field, outlined by the "ring fibers" of the basement membrane. The reticular fibers in the cords form a meshwork. In the human spleen the reticular fibers of the cords, as seen well between the upper two sinuses, form a collar or circlet around the sinus. The reader is referred to Koboth's work for additional valuable reconstructions of red pulp. (From Koboth, E. 1939. Beitr. Pathol. Anat. 103:11.)

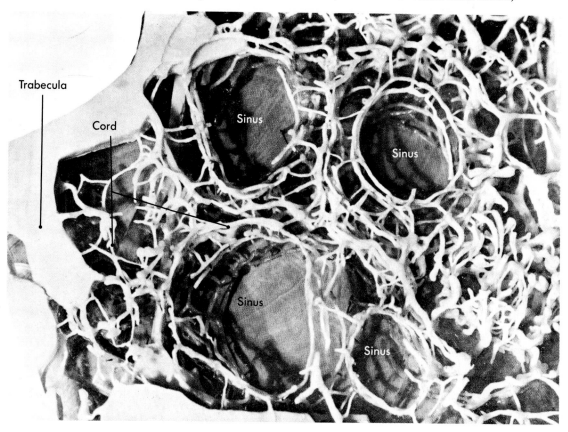

Trabecula

Cord

Sinus

Sinus

Sinus

Sinus

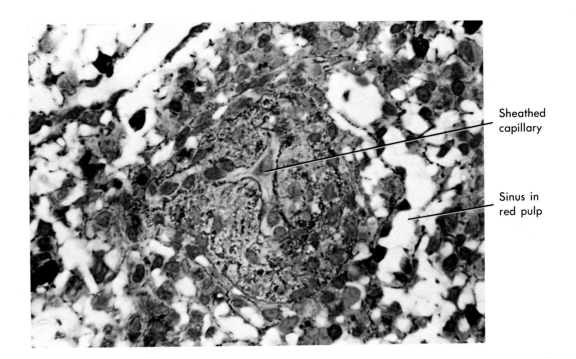

Sheathed
capillary

Sinus in
red pulp

16–20 Spleen of a dog, red pulp. In this light
micrograph, an arterial vessel, which is
actually a capillary, bifurcates within the sheath. Its
endothelium is high, effacing the lumen. The sheath
consists of phagocytes with strands of extracellular
reticulum running between them. The sheath is about
75 μm in diameter. The surrounding red pulp
contains sinuses. The darkly stained free cells in the
red pulp are granulocytes. One, in the left upper
corner of the field, is crossing the wall of a sinus.
Erythrocytes, which abound in red pulp, are
unstained in this preparation. PAS-hematoxylin stain.
× 650. (From Weiss, L. 1962. Am. J. Anat. 111:131.)

the walls of venous vessels. Thus, by correlating
their two sets of observations, the McCuskeys
concluded that the circulation through the red
pulp of the spleen is anatomically open.

Snook, who provided evidence for an open
circulation in many spleens, found that in some
species, notably the guinea pig, arterial capillaries appeared to connect directly with venous
vessels. However, his conclusion was based on
silvered preparations, which stain extracellular
material—specifically, basement membrane and
reticular fibers. Endothelium and other cellular
structures are not revealed, and it may not be
possible to differentiate an arterial terminal that

widely separated from veins; and the walls of the
veins, as seen by electron microscopy, contain
apertures that open to the pulp spaces. It is
hardly possible that such a spleen has an anatomically closed vascular bed, yet Knisely described the circulation as closed. In a sophisti-
cated and fastidious study the McCuskeys
correlated their observations on the living circulation, made using cool intense xenon light and
recorded by motion picture, with fixed and sectioned spleen studies by electron microscopy.
They found that blood flows out of arterial capillary terminations into the reticular meshwork
of red pulp. However, in this reticular meshwork
the blood is channeled by the cytoplasmic processes of reticular cells, which may form tubular
structures. These channels convey the blood to

16–21 Portion of a periarterial macrophage sheath.
The arterial capillary at the center of the
sheath (upper left corner) has a triangular shape
because of oblique sectioning. Endothelial cells (E_a)
impinge on the red cell in the lumen. A sinus (**S**)
filled with red cells delimits the periphery of the
sheath. Macrophages (**M**) containing ingested material
are packed tightly into the sheath reticulum. Note the
lucent centers in many residual bodies (**arrowheads**).
Basement membrane outlines the arterial capillary and
forms a broken line beneath the row of transversely
sectioned sinus endothelial cells (E_s) at the bottom of
the field. Reticular fibers of the same dense material
run through the sheath and surround reticular cells
(**RC**). × 3,400. (From Blue, J., and Weiss, L. The
American Journal of Anatomy, 1981.)

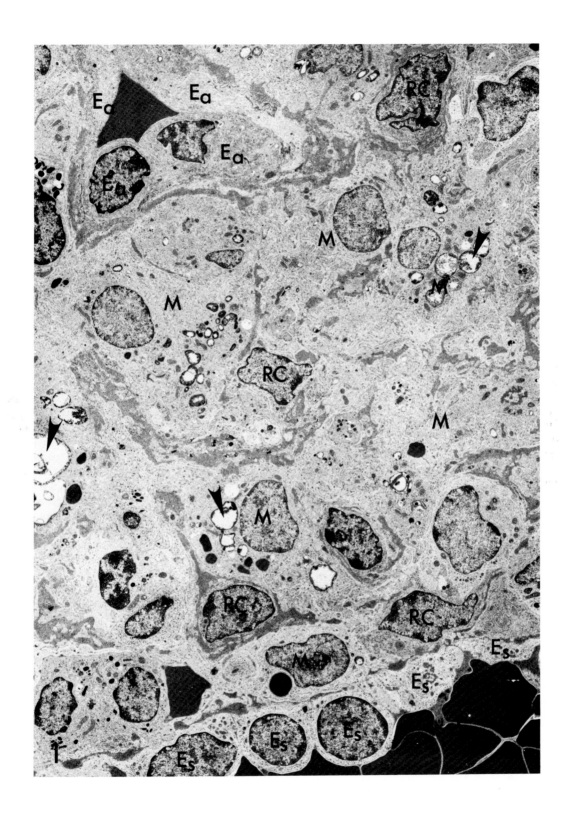

lies near a venous vessel from one that has actual endothelial continuity with a vein.

A number of scanning electron-microscopic studies have been done on casts of the spleen's vasculature. The casts have been made by injecting liquid plastic into splenic blood vessels, allowing it to harden, and then digesting away the tissue. Some investigators have concluded that the vasculature is open; others, that the vasculature is closed. With this technique, however, it is difficult to differentiate streams of plastic that had been enclosed by blood vessels from those that had not. Again, as in silver impregnation techniques for reticulum, this method does not seem suitable for determining whether the vascular bed of the spleen is anatomically open or closed.

In an ingenious approach to the question, Chen administered microspheres 3 to 4 μm in diameter intravenously to rabbits and found a portion of the spheres in the lumen of splenic sinuses. He concluded that there were some direct connections of arterial vessels to sinuses because, on the basis of earlier electron-microscopic observations of blood cell passage in the spleen, he believed that the interendothelial slits of vascular sinuses could not open wide enough to let through microspheres this large. However, intraendothelial slits 5 to 6 μm wide have been reported by Thomas in dog spleen perfused under physiological conditions. It appears, moreover, from Toghill and Prichard's work that spherocytes (spherical red blood cells larger than 3–4 μm in diameter) can cross the interendothelial slits of vascular sinuses with pressure generated by norepinephrine. Thus, the inference that interendothelial slits cannot open wide enough to allow microspheres 3 to 4 μm to pass through lacks sufficient experimental support.

Because there is an anatomically open vascular bed in the red pulp of the spleen, it must not be assumed that blood flow is delayed, irregular, or inefficient. A number of studies using red cells labeled with chromium-51 indicate that 98 to 99% of the blood entering human spleen flows through it in about 30 sec. In the spleen of dogs and cats, however, a component of the circulating blood passes through more slowly, indicating that these spleens have a reservoir function for erythrocytes. Groom and colleagues have carried out a kinetic analysis of red cell washout from perfused isolated spleens and have identified three functional compartments of blood flow in cat spleen. The first compartment offers fast flow. It receives 90% of total splenic blood flow and has a transit time of 30 sec, comparable to that of skeletal muscle. With respect to this fast compartment, the spleen may be said to have a circulation that is anatomically open and physiologically closed. It is likely that efficient blood flow is accomplished through the reticular meshwork of the red pulp by the formation of tubular conduits made of the sheetlike processes of reticular cells. A second compartment demonstrated by Song and Groom has an intermediate flow. It receives 9% of blood flow and has a transit time of 8 min. This compartment accounts for the blood-storage capacity of cat spleen and largely disappears when the spleen is induced to contract and expel the stored blood cells. The last compartment is slow, handling approximately 1% of blood flow with a transit time of 1 h. This compartment contains reticulocytes and perhaps some granulocytes that are held in the spleen for a short time to finish their maturation before they are released to the general circulation.

In conclusion, the circulation of the spleen is anatomically open where blood passes from arterial endings through the reticular meshwork and then into venous sinuses or veins. There does appear to be some variation in blood pathway, since the distance between arterial endings and venous walls may vary and the contents of the meshwork through which blood passes may include variable amounts of macrophages, hematopoietic cells, stored blood cells, plasma, etc. These anatomical arrangements in red pulp offer several types of flow. The principal flow is rapid, as rapid as that through other organs. But there is also (in some, but not in human spleens) a significant storage compartment, as well as a compartment that allows developing blood cells to finish their maturation. The reader is referred to the papers of Blue and Weiss for a full discussion of the splenic circulation.

Blood Processing

Plasma is separated from blood cells in the splenic circulation so that the cells are highly concentrated in red pulp, as shown both by direct puncture of the spleen and by microscopic study of the living circulation. The mechanism of separation depends on contraction of the splenic vein after sympathetic nerve stimulation, forcing plasma out of veins and vascular sinuses. The plasma crosses the spleen, is taken up by the deep lymphatics, and is carried out of the spleen to the thoracic duct. Barcroft and Poole abolished the spleen's capacity to remove plasma by cutting its vasomotor nerves. Concentration of blood cells in the spleen enhances its storage function. In animals with a muscular capsule, such as dogs and cats, a reserve mass of blood cells may be rapidly reintroduced into the circulation when adrenergic stimulation causes massive capsular contraction.

The spleen monitors circulating erythrocytes. It permits viable cells to pass through rapidly but detains and destroys or modifies damaged or aged erythrocytes. These functions are carried out in red pulp. The cords of sinusal spleens and the pulp spaces of nonsinusal spleens that consist of a reticular meshwork loaded with macrophages pose hazards to erythrocytes. Erythrocytes discharged into this meshwork from arterial terminations must travel through it in order to exit via the vascular sinuses and veins. The interstices of the meshwork are rather fine; when filled with bulky macrophages, they are even finer, and erythrocytes must be quite pliant to squeeze through. As an erythrocyte ages, it becomes more fragile and less apt to survive this cordal pathway. Indeed, the oxygen tension and the cholesterol and glucose concentrations of the cords make erythrocytes more rigid by affecting their hemoglobin, plasma membrane, and energy-producing capacity. This red cell conditioning may push a marginally viable erythrocyte toward phagocytosis. The unshielded presence of macrophages in the cordal pathway, moreover, not only places passing erythrocytes in direct range of these phagocytes but gives the extracellular fluids a high concentration of hydrolytic enzymes, which are secreted by the macrophages and bathe the cells in passage. An aged erythrocyte will lose sialic acid on its surface, exposing galactose residues. The spleen may recognize these galactose moieties, cause such erythrocytes to pool in the reticular meshwork, and phagocytize them. Passing through the interendothelial slit of vascular sinuses also constitutes a test for erythrocyte viability. Erythrocytes must be pliant to slip through the interendothelial slits. Rigid erythrocytes, like those in congenital spherocytic anemia, become "hung up" in the interendothelial slits and pool in the reticular meshwork, outside the vascular sinuses. Pliant erythrocytes that contain rigid inclusions, such as parasitic malarial organisms, may have the rigid inclusion "pitted out" at the sinus wall. The pliant portion of the erythrocyte passes through the interendothelial slit while the rigid portion is held back. The pliant portion then snaps off; it enters the lumen of the sinus and thence the circulation as a smaller erythrocyte that tends to be spherical. The rigid part remains behind and is typically phagocytized by macrophages lying against the outside surface of the walls of vascular sinuses.

Monocytes of the blood passing through the spleen are selectively removed from the circulation and sequestered in the white pulp, the marginal zone, and the red pulp, where they may rapidly undergo conversion into macrophages. Large numbers of macrophages derived in this manner are always present in the spleen and are responsible for its great phagocytic capacity. In malaria and in other processes involving the reaction and enlargement of the spleen, the spleen appears to release humoral substances that induce the bone marrow to produce and release more monocytes. These cells come to the spleen and considerably augment its population of macrophages.

B and T cells of the recirculating lymphocyte pool enter the spleen and follow distinctive pathways, as determined experimentally in rodents. They are first distributed through red pulp and the marginal zone. Many go right on out of the spleen by way of veins, but a significant fraction migrates through the reticular meshwork into white pulp. T cells enter the periarterial lymphatic sheaths and move around there for approximately 4 to 6 h, whereas B cells enter lymphatic nodules and stay there for a somewhat longer time. T and B cells may engage in antibody production as discussed in the next section, but if they do not, they leave the spleen via efferent lymphatics or veins to continue migrating as part of the recirculating lymphocytic pool.

Granulocytes may also be stored in the spleen. Moreover, in the rat, eosinophils, which differentiate primarily in bone marrow, are released to the spleen for final maturation before they enter the general circulation. Approximately one-third of the platelets of the body are normally stored in the spleen in ready reserve, even in spleens like the human that lack a reservoir function for erythrocytes. Under certain pathological conditions, platelets may be trapped in the spleen with such avidity that there are too few in the circulation, and bleeding results. Similarly, the spleen may remove slightly damaged but functionally competent erythrocytes with such zeal that an anemic crisis is precipitated. These con-

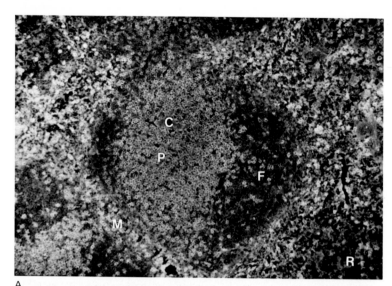

A

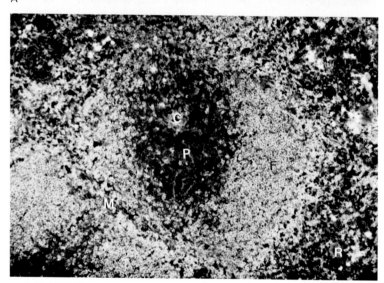

B

16–22 Spleen, mouse. Distribution of T and B lymphocytes as revealed by fluorescence immunocytochemistry. T and B cells are specifically stained in these frozen sections by a technique dependent on antibodies to the surface of T and B cells, respectively. The antibody is conjugated to a fluorescent marker, visible by fluorescence microscopy. In **A,** the central artery **(C)** is surrounded by the periarterial lymphatic sheath **(P),** which is stained by the anti-T-cell reagent, whereas the lymphatic nodule in the field **(F)** is largely unstained. The marginal zone **(M)** is stained. **R,** red pulp. Thus T lymphocytes are concentrated in the periarterial lymphatic sheath and marginal zone. In **B,** B lymphocytes are stained. Here the lymphatic nodule **(F)** and the marginal zone **(M)** are stained. Thus B lymphocytes are concentrated in lymphatic nodules and are largely absent from the periarterial lymphatic sheath. Both T and B cells are present in the marginal zone. See text and see Fig. 15–19 for distribution of T and B lymphocytes in lymph nodes (From Weissman, I. L. 1975. Transpl. Rev. 24:159.)

ditions, typically associated with a large spleen and designated *hypersplenism*, may be cured by splenectomy.

The capacity of the spleen to clear materials from the blood may be estimated by tagging test substances with radioactive isotopes and injecting them intravascularly. With this method it is possible to determine both the rate at which the isotope accumulates in the spleen (as inferred in human beings by counting radioactivity over the left upper quadrant of the abdomen) and the rate at which radioactivity disappears from the blood. Although lungs, liver, bone marrow, and other reticuloendothelial tissues also clear blood of particulate material, it is likely that the spleen's clearance capacity per gram of tissue is greatest.

Antibody Production

The spleen efficiently traps lymphocytes, monocytes, and antigen from the blood and permits them to interact and produce antibody. Antigen is first trapped and then phagocytized by macrophages in the marginal zone and red pulp. It subsequently moves into white pulp and surrounds lymphatic nodules, thereby lying at the junction of T- and B-cell zones (Fig. 16–22). Within the white pulp, antigen may be retained on the surface of antigen-presenting cells and macrophages.

In a primary immune response, antibody-producing cells appear first within the periarterial lymphatic sheaths as part of clusters of 20 to 100 or more cells. The cells migrate to the periphery of the sheaths and, at the same time, proliferate and secrete antibody. Then, traveling by routes that are not fully understood, they appear in red pulp as mature plasma cells and accumulate there. In secondary immune responses and in many primary responses that persist, germinal centers form and, as in lymph nodes, augment the antibody response and increase the number of memory cells.

References and Selected Bibliography

General

Barcroft, J., and Poole, L. T. 1927. The blood in the spleen pulp. J. Physiol. Lond. 64:23.

Blue, J., and Weiss, L. 1981a. Periarterial macrophages sheaths (ellipsoids) in cat spleen-an electron microscope study. Am. J. Anat. 161:115.

Crosby, E. H. 1959. Normal functions of the spleen relative to red blood cells: A review. Blood 14:399.

Fujita, T. 1974. A scanning electron microscope study of the human spleen. Arch. Histol. Jpn. 37:187.

Irino, S., Murkami, T., Fujita, T., Nagatani, T., and Kaneshige, T. 1978. Microdissection of tannin-osmium impregnated specimens in the scanning electron microscope: Demonstration of arterial terminals in human spleen. In O. Johari and R. P. Becker (eds.), Scanning Electron Microscopy/1978, pt. II. Chicago: SEM, Inc., p. 111.

Pereira, G. P. 1978. Evidence for a blood splenic white pulp barrier using a biologically inert electron-opaque tracer. In Johari and R. P. Becker (eds.), Electron Microscopy/1978, pt. II. Chicago: SEM, Inc. p. 649.

Pictet, R., Orci, L., Forssmann, W. B., and Girardier. 1969. An electron microscope study of the perfusion-fixed spleen. I. The splenic circulation and the RES concept. Z. Zellforsch. Mikrosk. Anat. 96:372.

Snook, T. 1950. A comprehensive study of the vascular arrangements in mammalian spleens. Am. J. Anat. 87:31.

Weiss, L. 1974. A scanning electron microscopic study of the spleen. Blood 43:665.

Circulation

Bjorkman, S. E. 1947. The splenic circulation with special reference to the function of the spleen sinus wall. Acta Med. Scan. 128 (Suppl. 191): 7.

Chen, L. T. 1978. Microcirculation of the spleen: An open or closed circulation? Science (Wash, D.C.) 201:157.

Groom, A. C., and Song, S. H. 1962. Effects of norepinephrine on washout of red cells from the spleen. Am. J. Physiol. 221:255.

Groom, A. C., Song, S. H., Lim, O., and Campling, B. 1971. Physical characteristics of red cells collected from the spleen. Can. J. Physiol. Pharmacol. 49:1092.

Irino, S., Murkami, T., and Fujita, T. 1977. Open circulation in the human spleen. Dissection scanning electron microscopy of conductive-stained tissue and observation of resin vascular casts. Arch. Histol. Jpn. 40:297.

Knisely, M. H. 1936. Spleen studies. I. Microscopic observations of the circulatory system of living unstimulated mammalian spleen. Anat. Rec. 65:23.

MacKenzie, D. W., Whipple, A. O., and Wintersteiner, M. P. 1941. Studies on the microscopic anatomy and physiology of living transilluminated mammalian spleens. Am. J. Anat. 68:397.

MacNeal, W. J. 1929. The circulation of blood through the spleen pulp. Arch. Pathol. Lab. Med. 7:215.

Mall, F. P. 1902. The circulation through the pulp of the dog's spleen. Am. J. Anat. 2:316.

McCuskey, R. S., and McCuskey, P. A. 1977. In vivo microscopy of the spleen. Bibl. Anat. 16:121.

Erythrocytes

Crosby, W. H. 1977. Splenic remodeling of red cell surfaces. Blood 50:643.

Lux, S. E., and John, K. M. 1977. Isolation and partial characterization of a high molecular weight red cell membrane protein complex normally removed by the spleen. Blood 50:625.

Song, S. H., and Groom, A. C. 1971b. The distribution of red cells in the spleen. Can. J. Physiol. Pharmacol. 49:734.

Song, S. H., and Groom, A. C. 1972. Sequestration and possible maturation of reticulocytes in the normal spleen. Can. J. Physiol. Pharmacol. 50:400.

Weiss, L., and Tavassoli, M. 1970. Anatomical hazards to the passage of erythrocytes through the spleen. Semin. Hematol. 7:372.

Immune Responses

Mitchell, J., and Abbot, A. 1971. Antigens in immunity. XVI. A light and electron microscope study of antigen localization in the rat spleen. Immunology 21:207.

Nossal, G. J. V., Austin, C. M., Pye, J., and Mitchell, J. 1966. Antigens in immunity. XII. Antigen trapping in the spleen. Int. Arch. Allergy 29:368.

Innervation

Heusermann, U., and Stutte, H. J. 1977. Electron microscopic studies of the innervation of the human spleen. Cell Tissue Res. 184:225.

Kudoh, G., Hoshi, K. and Murkami, T. 1979. Fluorescence microscopic and enzyme histochemical studies of the innervation of the human spleen. Arch. Histol. Jpn. 42:169.

Lymphocytes

Ford, W. L., and Smith, M. E. 1978. Lymphocyte recirculation between the spleen and blood. In Role of the Spleen in the Immunology of Parasitic Diseases. Tropical Diseases Research Series No. 1. Basel, Switzerland: Schwabe and Co. A.G., p. 29.

Mitchell, J. 1973. Lymphocyte circulation in the spleen. Marginal zone bridging channels and their possible role in cell traffic. Immunology 24:93.

Marginal Zone

Blue, J., and Weiss, L. 1981c. Species variations in the structure and function of the marginal zone: An electron microscope study of the cat spleen. Am. J. Anat. 161:169.

Sasou, S., Satodate, R., and Katsura, S. 1976. The marginal sinus in the perifollicular region of the rat spleen. Cell Tissue Res. 172:195.

Pathology

Bowdler, A. J. 1975. The spleen and haemolytic disorders. Clin. Haematol. 4:231.

Weiss, L. 1979. The spleen. In Role of the Spleen in the Immunology of Parasitic Diseases. Tropical Diseases Research Series No. I. Basel, Switzerland: Schwabe and Co. A.G., p. 7.

Red Pulp

Blue, J., and Weiss, L. 1981b. Vascular pathways in non-sinusal red pulp: An electron microscope study of cat spleen. Am. J. Anat. 161:135.

Chen, L. T., and Weiss, L. 1972. Electron microscopy of the red pulp of human spleen. Am. J. Anat. 134:425.

Chen, L. T., and Weiss, L. 1973. The role of the sinus wall in the passage of erythrocytes through the spleen. Blood 41:529.

Song, S. H., and Groom, A. C. 1971a. Storage of blood cells in the spleen of the cat. Am. J. Physiol. 220:779.

White Pulp

Galindo, B., and Imaeda, T. 1962. Electron microscope study of the white pulp of the mouse spleen. Anat. Rec. 143:399.

Satodate, R., Ogasawara, S., Sasou, S., and Katsura, S. 1971. Characteristic structure of the splenic white pulp of rats. J. Reticuloendothel Soc. 10:428.

Snook, T. 1946. Deep lymphatics of the spleen. Anat. Rec. 94:43.

Veerman, A. J. O., and van Ewijk, W. 1975. White pulp in the spleen of rats and mice. A light and electron microscopic study of lymphoid and non-lymphoid cell types in T- and B-areas. Cell Tissue Res. 156:417.

Weiss, L. 1974. The white pulp of the spleen. The relationships of arterial vessels, reticulum and free cells in the periarterial lymphatic sheath. Bull. Johns Hopkins Hosp. 115:99.

Index